Supermodels'
beauty
secrets

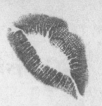

Supermodels' beauty

secrets

hot tips for style, beauty and fashion
from the world's top models

Victoria Nixon

PIATKUS

Copyright © 2002 by Victoria Nixon

First published in 2002 by
Judy Piatkus (Publishers) Limited
5 Windmill Street,
London W1T 2JA

email: info@piatkus.co.uk

The moral right of the author has been asserted

A catalogue record for this book is available from the British Library

ISBN 0 7499 2344 X

Text design by Goldust Design
Edited by Louise Crathorne

This book has been printed on paper manufactured with respect
for the environment using wood from managed sustainable resources

Data manipulation by Phoenix Photosetting, Chatham, Kent
Printed and bound in Great Britain by
Bookmarque Ltd, Mitcham, Surrey

Contents

Acknowledgements

I was asked to write this book because of my experiences in the modelling world, so I must thank a few people who encouraged my career.

Thanks to singer Paul Jones, who spotted me in school uniform, in the depths of Yorkshire, when he was on tour with his band Manfred Mann, and convinced me that London would be more my cup of tea, when I left school.

Thank you to the fashion photographers I particularly enjoyed working with – Richard Avedon, Arthur Elgort and Helmut Newton – whose work I still admire today.

And many thanks to my English agent and dear friend, Jill Rushton, who was always, and still is, a caring, protective mother-figure and confidante to her many girls.

I'm also grateful to have had the opportunity to hang out with my heroes Salvador Dali and Andy Warhol and a handful of rock stars (you know who you are) who longed to teach me bad habits but never succeeded!

The Book

....

I want to thank all the models who contributed their secrets and tips, for their time and thoughtful answers to my endless questions.

I couldn't have written this book without knowing my shop was in good hands – so thank you Shelley and Agnieszka for working so hard and ensuring we continue to sell the most delicious sandwiches in London.

Huge thanks to Alice Davis, my editor at Piatkus, for her enthusiasm, patience and encouragement. Every first-time author needs an editor like Alice.

And lastly, my heart-felt thanks to my partner Michael for his invaluable help in all areas of making this book a reality – it's dedicated to you.

Introduction

Jerry, Helena, Naomi, Claudia, Christy, Cindy, Linda, Elle and Kate – surnames not required. We all know the girls who transformed the image of models from coat-hangers and rock star appendages into multi-national enterprises better known than the products and designers they promote.

And the tradition continues with the more recent girls – Liberty Ross, Jodie Kidd, Catherine Hurley and Sophie Dahl – surnames an asset, who continue to put the super into supermodel by skilfully appearing to make incredible levels of beauty seem attainable to every woman with a credit card.

In an age when the worldwide female population are spending more time and money on beauty care than ever before, I thought it an appropriate moment to take a look at the beauty secrets of the true female icons of the twenty-first century and to discover the reasons they continue to look so timelessly 'right'.

How is it possible for a supermodel's skin to always glow and her hair to shine when she spends half her life on planes?

And how does she keep her shape so effortlessly? Why doesn't she ever look stressed? Why is she always so effortlessly stylish? She must spend a fortune on skin-care products.

The truth will surprise you. Only a small part of a super-model's 'off-duty' life is devoted to her looks. She doesn't work out all day; she doesn't wear designer clothes head-to-toe – and her bathroom cupboard is not jammed with expensive 'miracle' creams.

For ten years I was an international model working in Paris, Milan, London and New York. I was discovered by photographer Helmut Newton whilst gazing longingly at a pair of purple suede boots that I yearned for, but couldn't afford in a Bond Street (London) shop window. He subsequently photographed me for *Vogue*, giving me my entrée into the world of fashion that was to be my learning curve for a decade. During my time as a model I worked with many of the world's most talented photographers, fashion editors, make-up artists and stylists whilst they created their innovative and exciting editorial and advertising campaigns, to which I enthusiastically contributed. This proved to be invaluable experience for my future careers of stylist, beauty editor and fashion writer.

I also worked with some of the most beautiful cover-girls in the world from whom I discovered a strange and fascinating paradox – the more spectacular a woman looks, the simpler her beauty and fashion regime.

I observed that the real stunners have a nonchalance and sensuality that doesn't come from expensive jars of cream, but from the realisation that there is more to life than the way they look.

Okay, I know what you're thinking. It's easy to be nonchalant when you look naturally wonderful, but the attitude of these girls is not borne of a belief that they're above needing help, but from an insight and realistic knowledge learned through their work, of the limitations and expectations of beauty and hair products, diet, exercise and clothes.

Most supermodels will tell you that before they began their careers, they didn't rate a second glance in the local pub, and their best friend at school won all the beauty prizes. Supermodels are usually the first to admit their 'look' was unimpressive before a professional with a keen eye saw their potential when they were gauche and gangly – and the metamorphosis began.

The transformation from beanpole to cover-girl owes a little to the original flesh and bones and a great deal to the experts hired for each job; that elite band of make-up artists, hairdressers and fashion stylists – and of course the fashion editors and photographers who invent and capture that final image of perfection.

Having constant, direct access to these experienced image makers gives supermodels a wealth of insider tips, trade secrets, advice and information about all aspects of their physical welfare. This unique insight remains invaluable for the rest of their lives. A top model will be recognised for her style and allure many years after she retires from the modelling world.

But it takes much more than a photogenic face to make it to the top. Any fashion photographer will tell you that the girls who make the best models are the ones with the right attitude – the smartest. If 'intelligent cover-girl' seems somewhat oxymoronic to you, consider the pressures of having to look your best **every day**; the resilience needed to travel the world alone; to be a team player on set and to always immediately understand what is expected of you in the big picture.

A girl will be booked time and time again if she's punctual, organised, gets on well with the client and crew, has good manners and a great sense of humour. All this counts as much as her ability to understand the camera angles and lighting.

To be focused; to have good strategies to cope with stress; to have your very own flair in order to deliver a flawless performance on a painstakingly tricky job **and** to make it all look easy and fun, takes a fair amount of self-discipline. It's not accidental that most supermodels become successful business women after their modelling careers are over.

There is no question that supermodels look like dreams, but their beauty and fashion routines are incredibly real and accessible. I asked some of the world's top models – both past and present – to help de-mystify and simplify their world and tell us what works and what doesn't.

In the 1950s, Fiona Campbell-Walter was the first ever British model to become as famous as a Hollywood movie star. Now Baroness Thyssen, she remains as stunning today as in her heyday.

Yet her beauty regimes are as simple as those of Catherine Hurley, the young Oxford medical undergraduate who is fast becoming the next hot supermodel – with

Jean Paul Gaultier, Max Factor and Renault car campaigns already under her belt.

Fiona, Catherine, Helena Christensen, and many more of our favourite supermodels, disclose and define their trade secrets and tips for beauty, style and attitude – to reveal the art of looking fabulous at all times without looking as though you've tried for a moment.

Part One
Face and Hair

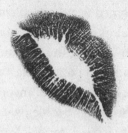

That carefree cover of your favourite glossy takes months to plan and can cost a thwacking great fortune to produce. Making sure the right girl for the job is available at the same time as the chosen photographer and his preferred team of make-up artist, stylist and hairdresser takes inspired planning.

It's vital that the selected supermodel shows up in the best possible condition – particularly her skin – which must be immaculate, glowing and smooth. Nothing reflects health and well-being more than a woman's complexion and models have to overcome many scary obstacles and pressures to ensure their skin is always vibrant.

The mantra for maintaining good skin used to be simple

– cleanse, tone and moisturise twice daily. The main problem now is making sense of the plethora of skin products swamping the market place, and ensuring the skin doesn't get overloaded.

It's easy to feel confused and bewildered by the constant bombardment of jars, tubes and bottles, each new one claiming to be the 'next big thing'. Even seasoned magazine beauty editors struggle to keep up with the billion dollar machine selling every conceivable option and lotion for every real and imagined beauty problem.

The supermodel is careful to simplify rather than complicate her skin-care regime to avoid overload. With so many beauty products containing 'active' ingredients around these days, it's so easy to unconsciously over-treat skin and cause unnecessary problems.

One of the first facts a model learns from make-up artists and dermatologists is to never assume that an expensive skin product must always be better than a cheap one. A small but expensive glass jar of cream containing a special ingredient (which may not be special at all) looks more convincing than a simple plastic container, but if you check the ingredients, there will be remarkable similarities.

So the most expensive products in the world are not always the best but it is important to be astute about purchasing products that suit the type of skin they were made for.

1

The secrets of glowing skin

Cleanse, tone and moisturise is what we're all taught to do, right? Sounds simple enough but it's staggering – no horrifying – how many women (including aspiring models) use the wrong products on their skin, often clogging their pores with over-rich creams or stripping valuable oils from their skin by using an alcohol based preparation as a facial toner.

A Simple Cleanse

Cleaning the skin properly is the most important favour you can do for your complexion but too much cleansing, even with just water, can wash away the skin's naturally produced oils, making it dry and irritated. Cleansers come in many forms ranging from bars and gels to lotions, scrubs and creams and it's vital to use the right form of cleanser for your skin, which should always be determined by your skin type (see chart on page 16)

After you've applied your correct cleanser, it should be gently massaged in with the fingers and left on for a minute to allow make-up to melt away. This will make it easier to sweep away dirt, pollution and cosmetic build-up without tugging at the skin. Do this process twice or until your tissue/cotton wool/facial cloth has no trace of dirt.

It's important to remember to take the old slap off every night however tired or drunk you are. No excuses – well maybe one – if you happen to find yourself in bed with someone new and you're not ready to expose the 'raw' you. But hopefully, this situation won't occur too often, otherwise the dilemma could be more about old slapper than old slap!

Never use a cleanser with exfoliant properties every day. It can scratch the living layer of skin. If you want to use a facial scrub regularly, look for one with synthetic granules that won't scratch the skin and never exfoliate more than three times a week.

Tone it down!

Toners are designed to refresh the skin after cleansing but I think they're the most misunderstood part of the skin-care regime and, in my experience, often do more harm than good. Using a toner that is too strong for your skin-type will strip it of natural oils. If your skin is taut after toning, and quickly becomes excessively oily, it's trying too hard to over-compensate and you're using the wrong product.

Many models told me they'd had so many bad experiences with toners, that now they simply don't use them and thoroughly cleanse their face twice instead. Most toners contain alcohol which, in my experience, is better poured down the throat than put on the face. There are three types of toners available:

1. Skin Fresheners. The mildest, contains more water than alcohol.

2. Clarifying Lotions. These contain more alcohol than water plus other chemical agents to remove the top layer of dead skin.

3. Astringents. These rely totally on alcohol (arrghhh!) to remove traces of dirt.

If you still feel you need a gentle toner to refresh your skin, ask your chemist to make up one of the following:

■ Normal to Dry Skin. ⅔ distilled water and ⅓ witch hazel.

■ Normal to Greasy Skin. ⅔ rose water and ⅓ witch hazel.

■ Sensitive Skin. Rose water and distilled water in equal quantities.

The 'no bull' moisturiser

It's simply an oil or cream designed to stop dehydration and act as a barrier against external elements. So why is it so difficult to find the right moisturiser when the market is saturated with them? Well that's the point. Too much choice without understanding the possibilities and limitations of the products available.

Models are able to short-circuit the confusing trawl around the department store cosmetic counters by accessing knowledge from the beauty editors and make-up artists they work with.

Of the thousands of new beauty products released into the market place every year, only one or two will possibly be worth changing from your current brand for. But how do you tell which are genuinely revolutionary and make a difference?

Magazines are not always reliable sources of information as they may endorse new products to keep their influential advertisers happy. The enormous advertising budgets of the multi-national cosmetics corporations are an essential part of the fashion magazine's revenue.

There's often a lot of pseudo-science on the packaging of moisturisers to impress and baffle us but the basic ingredients of a successful moisturiser are very simple – water, emollient to keep the water in, a humectant which absorbs and retains water, and maybe some kind of sun protection. Perfumes, preservatives and other ingredients may enhance the cosmetic elegance and chemical ability of the product.

'I believe in moisturising a lot, especially when I travel on planes, but I don't have a particular brand of skin-care that I stick with. I love trying out products from small, interesting shops because they smell wonderful or have a great texture. I just buy what I like at the time. It doesn't have to be expensive.'

Helena Christensen

What moisturisers can and can't do

- When you smooth a moisturiser onto your skin, the water evaporates, leaving the oil on the surface of the skin making it more supple and hydrated. This all happens at surface level. No moisture crosses into cells or goes into deep layers of skin.

- A moisturiser's main job is to provide an additional protection shield to retain the moisture that is already in the skin. The hydration of the skin occurs deep in its lower layers where no moisturiser can penetrate.

- A good moisturiser will stay on top of the skin, not sink in. And the more oils a moisturiser has, the more effective it will be in preventing loss of moisture from the skin. The more water the skin retains, the younger and more supple it feels, therefore the function of a good moisturiser is to slow the rate at which water is lost from the skin.

So choosing the right moisturiser for you is purely what reacts best on your skin. A good cream should be easy to smooth in and leave a film on the skin like a fine denier stocking rather than a pair of support tights – silky rather than greasy. Too much oil left on the surface may cause spots; too little will not plump up the dryness.

KNOW YOUR SKIN TYPE AND WHAT TO DO WITH IT

Skin Type	Characteristics	Always Use	Never Use
No Problem Skin	■ Always perfectly hydrated at deep and surface levels. ■ Firm and elastic.	■ Cleansing cream or lotion twice a day. ■ A mild freshener with no alcohol. ■ A mild oil-based moisturiser. ■ A night cream but only on rough, dry patches. ■ A non-drying mask once every two weeks to stimulate circulation.	■ Soap, detergent based products or abrasive cleanser.
Dry Skin	■ Is taut and dull with thin lines around the mouth and eyes.	■ Non-detergent neutral pH products. ■ Mineral water only to tone your face. ■ Cream for double cleansing. ■ An oil-based foundation. ■ An anti-wrinkle mask frequently.	■ Tap water or hot water.

Skin Type	Characteristics	Always Use	Never Use
Oily Skin	■ A shiny nose, forehead and chin. ■ Dilated pores, poor elasticity and a thick grain. This change of texture is what distinguishes a truly oily skin from an essentially normal skin that happens to have oily patches.	■ A lightly medicated soap used with mineral water (not tap water) or an anti-bacterial cleansing lotion two or three times a day. ■ Astringent in the morning only. ■ Use a milder astringent at night. ■ Use a clarifying mask once a week. ■ Use a professional deep-cleanse often.	■ Heavy cleansing creams. ■ Hot water or hard scrubbing. ■ Strong astringents.

Check sell-by dates and throw away anything that has changed colour, developed a smell or if a clear liquid becomes cloudy. These are strong indications that mould, fungi or bacteria are breeding in the product.

The truth about sun protection factors (SPFs)

For the past few years, skin-care companies have used the mantra 'SPF 15 moisturiser every day, even in winter, even on a cloudy day' and they have recently added sunscreens to everything from lipsticks to concealers.

But the Head of Research and Development at Clarins concedes that,

> *'if you are exposed to the sun for less than an hour a day, going from your flat to the office in shadow, then you don't need an SPF. The skin has in-built defences and can tolerate some UV. If you wear a sunscreen every day, you are constantly putting chemicals onto your skin that are often unnecessary. Unless you live in a country where you are exposed to sun all the time, it's a bit like taking headache pills when you don't need them. And if your skin is sensitive, it can create chronic sensitivity'.*

I couldn't have put it better myself. It makes sense to say that daily protection should change with the season. In the northern hemisphere, use a day cream with an SPF 15 in summer to guard against incidental exposure. In autumn change to SPF 8. But wearing a high daily SPF in winter could be doing more harm than good as the skin needs sunlight in order to synthesise vitamin D.

If you live in the southern hemisphere, where the ozone layer is at its thinnest, then it makes sense to wear the highest SPF available, at all times. Avoiding skin cancer takes precedence over chemical overload.

Choosing the right product for the job

Know the difference between a formula for everyday use, where sun exposure is incidental, (these are skin products with added SPFs) and sun-care products designed for deliberate sun exposure.

Sun-care products contain 'broad-spectrum' protection (UVA and UVB) and are too greasy and heavy to be worn under make-up. Moisturisers containing an SPF rarely have UVB protection and are simply not strong enough to protect you from relentless sunbathing.

- Cosmetics packaging gets more sophisticated by the day. It's not always easy to tell the difference between skin-care and sun-care products so read the labels carefully.

- If your moisturiser contains an SPF, you don't need one in your foundation too. Chemical sunscreens work by being absorbed into the skin and too many penetrating chemicals adds up to unnecessary overload.

- Wearing a high daily SPF in winter isn't a good idea. As well as needing sunlight to synthesise vitamin D, it protects us against Seasonal Affective Disorder (SAD) and helps build strong bones and skin.

- Recognise and respect the sun's health giving properties, rather than always fearing them. Use common sense. If the weather forecast says rain all day, give your skin a sunscreen break.

'The sun makes me feel completely happy — I love it. Luckily I've inherited my mother's skin — she's Peruvian — which tans easily and doesn't burn. I think it's important to let your skin breathe and not to get too uptight about it and enjoy the elements. But be sensible.'

Helena Christensen

The giant cosmetic corporations spend millions of dollars a year improving the quality of skin-care products. But it's important to recognise the 'feel-good factor' and the major part it plays in the purchasing of these products.

That expensive jar of cream will undoubtedly look better on your bathroom shelf and probably smells more sophisticated. But it may be too rich for your skin. On the other hand the cheap jar may be a perfect balance for your skin, but doesn't have the 'feel-good' visual factor.

All supermodels use the Drugstore/Gucci principle for their skin-care. They mix and match good-value, simple products with the designer luxury items they feel are worth the extra money.

Favourites that don't cost a fortune

- Vaseline Lip Therapy
- Optrex Eye Dew Blue Eye Drops
- Nivea Cream
- Simple Fast Acting Cleansing Lotion
- Astral Moisturiser
- Body Shop Elderflower Eye Gel
- Pampers Baby Wipes (good for cleaning faces as well as babies' bottoms)

Skin-care products that can make a difference

GUERLAIN'S MIDNIGHT SECRET

'I put this on my skin before going to bed. It re-oxygenates and stimulates the skin while I sleep so that I wake up feeling radiant and it has the most incredible texture. An absolute must for those mornings after late nights.'

Sophie Dahl

SUNDARI LAVENDER MOISTURISER

*'I replace this with the Neem Night Cream when
my skin is particularly dry, and once a week I
use the Night Time Nourishing Oil as a luxurious,
rich mask and leave it on overnight. I also love
Sundari Camomile Eye Oil because it makes your
eyes look fantastic even after a late night.'*

Christy Turlington

DR HAUSCHKA ROSE CREAM MOISTURISER

*'The Rose Cream is the star of this great holistic
range. It has no preservatives or petro-chemi-
cals and it's made from petals harvested at
dawn to capture their full-force. And it smells
divine.'*

Jerry Hall

SK-11 FACIAL TREATMENT REPAIR C

*'I simply won't go anywhere without vitamin C
repair Serum.'*

Liberty Ross

The low down on eye creams

Eye creams simply contain the same ingredients as moisturisers but are lighter in texture. They may include
antioxidants, skin soothers and even light reducing
pigments to reduce eye shadows. They are worth trying
because the thinnest skin of all is around the eyes where
there are limited oils and less fat.

Never confuse the uses of eye creams and gels. Eye gels

are formulated to deflate bags and give a cooling, refreshing sensation but rarely claim to moisturise the skin. And never apply AHA or retinal creams close to the eyes unless specified for that use.

> **TIP** The answer to seriously baggy eyes, when nothing else will work, is a thin layer of haemorrhoid cream, gently applied to the bags. Leave for ten minutes, and then remove the residue with eye make-up remover. This little trick has saved many nightmare situations for make-up artists but should only ever be used in an emergency.

I agree with Liberty Ross about serums and won't go anywhere without mine either. I use *Capture Essential* by Christian Dior on my skin daily, before applying moisturiser, and I swear it makes a difference.

But I think it's important to avoid the danger of being seduced into thinking that any of these products can perform miracles, and neglecting or ignoring the other important elements that keep your skin healthy.

2

Face savers that really work

Having the right regime for the epidermis, the outer layer of skin, isn't enough to maintain a great complexion. It's also essential to improve the quality and structure of skin from the inside.

During a hectic work schedule, especially at the times of year the fashion designers present their collections, models get over-tired, don't always eat properly and can get physically and emotionally run down. Add to that the cigarette smoke, a diet that lacks nutrients (particularly antioxidants like vitamins C and E) sunlight and air pollution – and some extra help is badly needed.

At this time models treat the deep layer of inner skin, the dermis, to a combined 1000 gram vitamin C and zinc tablet every day. It revitalises the skin's structure and quality, and improves the skin's ability to hold in moisture – vital for glowing skin.

Remember that it's the way we treat our skin – not the ageing process – that 'ages' facial skin the most.

Why water is every model's best friend

A doctor friend of mine told me he can see from ten paces whether a woman is drinking enough water each day, purely from the condition of her skin – and in his opinion, water is the best moisturiser in the world. The bulk of the human body (70%) is water and it's now widely believed that dehydration is the main culprit responsible for poor-looking skin.

Throughout the day, water is the must-have accessory for all on or off-duty models, who traditionally carry bottles of still water, and avoid anything sparkling like the plague. They drink it because they know it flushes out toxins, the enemies of glowing skin, and it also stops them nibbling snacks as it suppresses the appetite.

There can't be a woman left in the country who isn't aware of the benefits of drinking two litres of water a day. But the idea of consuming a huge bottle can seem daunting and impractical.

> **TIP** Buy four half litre handbag sized plastic bottles of your favourite still mineral water and dot them around the areas you frequent the most – desk, kitchen worktop, handbag, car, next to the TV and bed. Take a swig whenever you see a bottle. That way two litres a day won't seem so daunting.

When I first arrived in New York as a young, excitable model, my agent Eileen Ford offered me three pieces of advice. Eileen was at the helm of the Ford Model Agency, reputedly the most prestigious agency in the world at the time, representing household names like Jean Shrimpton, Lauren Hutton and Kim Basinger. So I thought I'd better listen.

Eileen's advice to me was to enjoy New York (easy), stay away from all illegal substances (harder), and to always start the day by drinking a glass of hot water. Just simple water, nothing added (boring).

I shrugged and persevered. To my utter amazement, I am still drinking a glass of hot water first thing every morning and have done so since those heady New York days. Little did I realise then that getting into hot water was the best beauty advice I have ever received. Don't add lemon juice – it's far too acidic for your system first thing, and make sure the water is not boiling but hotter than lukewarm. It's the heat and purity of the water that kick-starts your system like no other, cleansing and purifying your entire physical being.

Water works

- Drink before you get thirsty. Being thirsty means you're already dehydrated.

- Aim to drink eight glasses of still mineral water a day or more if you're exercising and another one for every cup of coffee, tea and alcohol.

- If you find two litres a day too much, work out the correct manageable quantity for your body by drinking one 8 fl oz glass of water per 20 lb of your body weight.

- Check if you're drinking the right amount of water by looking at the colour of your urine. The darker the colour, the more dehydrated you are. A light straw-colour is the perfect looking pee.

- Don't go mad and drink too much water. It can be counter-productive, diluting the minerals, including sodium, that your body needs.

Facts about facials

Off-duty models usually want to give their faces a rest – suffering from over-pampering fatigue – and they'll only succumb to a facial if they can be sure the facialist is the best around.

The quality of facials swerves dangerously from salon to salon. Many simply seem to be an expensive way of putting more creams on your face. A good facial is one you can't do yourself at home and makes you look positively glowing afterwards. In other words, someone with good exfoliating procedures and massaging skills, who will work out the condition of your skin and treat it accordingly (dehydrated, stressed etc) rather than giving the same facial every visit.

> *'I have tried many facials over the years, but the best person to give my complexion a boost is skin-care specialist Dr Michel Tordjam in Paris.'*
> *Elle Macpherson*

Kate Moss's current favourite is the Crystal Clear Oxygen facial, a new face treat from the United States available in the UK, Australia and most other large countries. More of a micro-dermabrasion treatment than a pure facial, the skin is exfoliated with a stream of fine mineral crystals which abrades (lightly sandblasts) dead cells and unplugs pores, smoothes surface lines and helps remove age spots.

The crystals and exfoliated layers of skin are then sucked away, stimulating the production of new cells and collagen in the deeper layers of the dermis. Jets of pure oxygen are then pumped onto the surface of the skin with a patent-pending puncture jet system that can actually penetrate the upper layers of cells – and finally the skin is fed vitamin-rich serums.

> *'I love Jo Malone facials and I regularly visit her when I'm in London. I prefer the natural approach to skin care, and her products really suit my sensitive skin type.'*   *Yasmin Le Bon*

Ask around for facial recommendations – word of mouth is always best. Failing that, ask about the training and experience of a facialist before you make an appointment. Enquire whether any instruments or machines are used during the facial and if so, what – and why?

Find out how much the facial costs and how long it takes. Also whether you need to let your skin 'breathe' afterwards or if you can slap on your make-up and go straight out.

You'll know when you've found someone who gives you the perfect facial just by looking in the mirror immediately afterwards. You shouldn't be blotchy or red and your skin should look instantly great.

Try to have a facial once a month. The skin's cells regenerate every 21 days, so it makes sense to get rid of the accumulation of dead cells. A good facial isn't cheap but is extremely beneficial and, for my money, takes precedence over manicures and all other treatments – apart from a good body massage!

How to make you own 'foodie' facials

The fridge is the place to look to find the best ingredients to pep up tired skin quickly:

- Mix a small pot of live yoghurt with the same amount of runny honey. Spread on face and leave for 15 minutes. Rinse with warm water; pat dry and apply lashings of moisturiser. (Best for normal skins)

- Mash an avocado with one teaspoon of lemon juice and two teaspoons of wheatgerm. Spread over face, avoiding eye area and leave for ten minutes. Rinse etc. (Best for dry skins)

■ Beat together an egg white and juice of half a lemon. Leave for ten minutes. Rinse etc. (Best for combination or oily skins)

Always cleanse your face before using a mask or you'll seal in the dirt rather than eliminating it – and avoid the eye area, especially the sensitive under-eye skin.

Be generous with the ingredients of your mask. They work best when laid on thick and when you're lying down, with your feet up, so that the body's oxygen all goes to your head, making the mask more effective.

After removing your mask, moisturise your face straight away so that your moisturiser can penetrate more deeply and be of maximum benefit.

Spot check

It's bad enough to have a nasty spot at any time, but pretty high on the Richter scale, if you're being paid a king's ransom to be photographed in close-up.

Know your spots. They come in three different types:

1. Comedones – blackheads and whiteheads caused by dead skin cells and excess oil. These spots love summer because heat and humidity cause perspiration and sunscreens trap oil. Use a PABA-free sunscreen and exfoliate often. Treat with Neutrogena Clear Pore Treatment.

> **TIP** Eye drops are a good emergency preventative treatment for open pores and blackheads as they contain a mild antiseptic.

2. Papular – the classic pink pimple. Caused when bacteria infect a clogged pore. Keep the face clean with bacteria-killing cleansers that have a benzoyl peroxide in them. Prescribed topical antibiotics or Differin gel help treat these best.

3. Vulgaris – acne, the most visual and complicated. Caused by over-active oil glands, abnormal cell turnover and an agitated inflammatory response. Treat with oral antibiotics that a dermatologist can prescribe. Do not cover unless absolutely necessary in which case use a medicated concealer like Clinique Anti-blemish Solution Conceale; Chin Breakout Relief by Joey New York; Laura Mercier Secret Camouflage or Trish McElvoy Concealer (supermodel favourite).

Some useful spot tips for you to bear in mind:

-   Never combine spot remedies.

-   Never squeeze unless absolutely necessary. It can leave scarring.

-   If spot demands emergency pop, remember the rule – pus, blood, pus. (The spot will return unless you get all the second lot of pus out.)

> **TIP** For emergency cover up, dab on any sort of astringent or alcohol, whether perfume, gin, or proper antiseptic. Then pat on concealer that isn't too dry or oily and a dab of powder.

3

Supermodel make-up tricks that last a lifetime

Most top models choose to wear no make-up when they're not working. It gives their skin time to breathe and relax. A pair of sunglasses and a dab of Vaseline on their lips does the job for that trip to the supermarket. When they're 'on show' this is how they achieve their 'natural' look.

The step-by-step guide to the perfect daytime face

Step 1 — Mirror

- Make sure your mirror (which should be large enough to see your entire outline down to your chest) is positioned very near a window with natural light.

Step 2 — Foundation

- Apply foundation carefully so that it doesn't begin or end anywhere. Dab and blend in lightly with your fingertips, paying special attention to the areas around the nostrils, eyes and where the face meets the neck.

- Your skin should still show through in a subtle way. If you can't see any facial contours, it's too heavy.

- There's no excuse, whatever your age, to have a face like a mask. These days foundations have hydrating properties and often contain light-diffusing ingredients, which disguise fine lines and give skin a dewy glow, rather than an ageing matte finish. Light reflective pigments help bounce light away from the skin, like tiny mirrors. The very latest foundations now offer 'photochromatic technology' which means they look totally natural in different lights, taking you from morning to evening.

- The best base to choose is a light, slightly moisturising formula in a shade that matches your own in any light.

- Make sure that if your moisturiser doesn't contain an SPF (sun protection factor), then your foundation does.

Step 3 — Concealer

- Apply concealer **after** foundation, otherwise the concealer will simply be rubbed off.

- Don't confuse traditional with highlighting concealers. A traditional concealer covers blemishes and is simply a thicker version of foundation. A highlighting concealer contains 'light-reflecting pigments', and tiny particles in the pigment refract light off the skin.

■ Use the concealer with the light-reflecting pigments to disguise dark circles under the eyes (not bags). Tilt your chin down slightly, and look up into the mirror. Apply and blend in the concealer gently. Never apply concealer to dark circles whilst looking straight into the mirror – you'll look like a panda.

■ If you don't have a traditional concealer to hand, use the dehydrated foundation that accumulates around the top of the tube or bottle – it's almost the same.

■ If you look tired and all the light-reflecting pigments in the world are failing you, brush a little matte (not sparkly) pink eyeshadow or blusher underneath the eyes. Sounds strange but it works.

Step 4 — Blusher

■ Always use a cream blusher in daylight for a younger, fresher look. Powders look 'cakey' and gels demand a perfect skin. Choose a blusher that's more pink than orange and avoid the ones with sparkly particles in daytime.

■ Dab on the blusher with your finger, blending in well. Smile when you apply it, so you get a good natural coverage on the apple of your cheek, gradually building up the colour. Check your side view to make sure there are no hard lines and finish off by dabbing a tiny amount at the bottom edge of the chin and on the eye socket.

■ Try applying blusher **before** your foundation for an even more natural look.

TIP To avoid unsightly lipstick marks on your glass, gently lick the edge of your glass where you intend to take a sip.

Step 5 — Powder

■ Forget about powder unless you have a very oily skin. Foundations these days 'set' themselves on the skin. They don't need powder to hold them. Apply an anti-shine product before your foundation to combat an oily forehead and chin.

Step 6 — Eyebrows

■ Eyebrows need to be groomed. Put some hairspray on a finger or brow brush and slick eyebrows into shape.

■ Never use a darker colour than your eyebrow shade and don't pluck them too thin.

■ Use a powder rather than a pencil and fill in the brow with a brush as opposed to drawing it in.

TIP Always pluck your eyebrows in the direction of the hair growth and pull the skin taut with your finger at the same time. Line up the beginning of your eyebrow with the inner corner of your eye and make sure the highest part of your arch lines up with the outer white of the eye. The first section of your brow leading up to the arch, should be the longest and the tail end, the shortest.

Step 7 — Eyeshadow

- Cover the entire eyelid, up to the browbone with a powder eyeshadow, slightly lighter than the skin above your eyes. This will undetectably open up the eyes making them look fresh and bright.

- Always choose shades of brown and grey for your main eyeshadow, in powder form to avoid creasing the socket. Remember it's not about colouring the eye but contouring it.

- Put the shade in an arch on the base of the brow bone.

- Dark shades make eyes recede; paler ones push them forward.

Step 8 — Eyeliner

- Treat eyeliner with a light hand, if you use it. Never use liquid liner underneath and on top of eyes.

■ When applying eyeliner to the upper lid, keep as close to the lashes as possible. If you're not too steady handed, rest your elbow on a hard surface while you sweep it along the lash line.

Step 9 — Mascara

■ Brush mascara over the top of the upper lashes, then twice from below.

> **TIP** Change your mascara when it gets dry and clunky. Every time you use the wand it pumps air into the case making it last less time than your other products.

Step 10 — Lips

■ Make thin lips fuller by applying a light-reflecting concealer around the outside of the lips and blend down into the lips themselves.

■ Use a lip pencil which matches your natural lip colour (*Spice* by Mac is the perfect lip colour for everyone) and outline your mouth just outside the lip-line. Never use a darker colour than your lips or you'll look like some Sixties joke.

■ Apply the lip colour inside the line with a lip brush and blend in with a pencil so there is no demarcation line. When choosing colour avoid anything that is dark and matte; these will make your mouth look small and pursed.

TIP No need to wipe it off and start again if you make a mess of your make-up. Make smudges and smears disappear with Shiseido's Eraser Pencil. Simply rub the tip over the mistake and it disappears.

- Light, medium and bright colours in sheer, dewy, glossy textures bring out the lips to full effect.

- For a natural, no lipstick effect that lasts all day, apply a lip stain, extending it slightly beyond the natural lip line.

- Take a natural coloured lip pencil and outline the mouth.

- Apply lip-gloss in a shiny pale colour to the centre of the lips only.

Make-up classics that will never date

Touche Eclat by Saint Laurent
This under-eye concealer with light-diffusing particles, pump action and built-in brush has been a favourite of Kate Moss and many others for years.

Fluid Sheers by Giorgio Armani
Already a favourite of Gisele and Naomi Campbell, this gives a fab, golden shimmer to skin – but go easy. Just one squirt.

Lipfinity by Max Factor

Eight-hour lip stain. Number 180 is the most natural lip-colour shade. So long lasting it has to be removed with eye make-up remover. 'Utterly bomb-proof', says Sheba Ronay.

Lip Pencil by Mac in Spice

Linda Evangelista was the first model to discover that Spice is the perfect natural colour for all lips. She wears it every single day and says it's simply perfect.

Aquablush by Chanel

This three-in-one product for lips, cheeks and eyes is Helena Christensen's favourite. 'She spent two minutes on her lips, eyes and cheeks with this product and looked better than when I'd spent an hour making her up!', says make-up artist Jonathan Malone.

Great Lash Mascara by Maybelline

This must-have mascara (200 million women users world-wide can't be wrong, including Christy Turlington and Eva Herzigova) never globs, separates beautifully and comes in five great shades. Shame about the pink and green wand though!

Eyelash Curler by Shu Uemura

There is hardly a model in the world who doesn't own a pair of these pinch-proof curlers. The supermodel trick is to use them before applying mascara, otherwise they stick to lashes.

Ten rules for evening beauty

It's easy to get carried away and to pile on the 'mood maquillage' without thinking it through. Bold and dramatic evening make-up can end up looking drag-queeny if you don't stick to these simple rules.

1. Base the colours you use for evening on those you use for the day and intensify them.

2. Focus on the lips or eyes – but not on both. Too tarty.

3. Use a primer under your foundation to keep the base in place all evening.

4. Don't confuse glow and shine. Use an anti-shine product under make-up on problem areas.

5. Anticipate the lighting to make sure you won't get caught out.

6. Use waterproof mascara and a lipstick-fixing product if you expect to be kissed and caressed.

7. Use eyeshadows with shimmer to catch the light.

8. If the focus is your eyes, remember the importance of blending well; no harsh lines.

9. If you're tanned, don't wear heavy make-up and especially not powder blusher.

10. Don't take your entire make-up bag for touch-ups. Choose multi-purpose, compact products instead.

4

Tressed for success.
The best hair tips ever

Our hair is a statement – just like our clothes and make-up. But somehow it's more important. A wonderful haircut gives us incredible confidence and a bad hair day makes us totally miserable.

The power our hair has over us lies in the fact that we have to put our faith in 'professionals' to create the look we want. If our chosen hair stylist, or colourist does a good job, we are in seventh heaven, but if they don't we leave the salon feeling wretched. We are putty in their hands!

Here's how to find the best cut, colour and haircare to ensure that going to a salon becomes a relaxing experience because you get what **you** want. The days of paying a fortune, going home, weeping and staying in for a week will be gone forever.

It's important to start with a hairstyle that suits you. It has to be in proportion with the rest of you, suit your face shape, enhance your clothes style, fit in with your lifestyle and say something about you.

Kate Moss completely transformed her career some time back when she suddenly appeared with a new urchin crop. So much so that it's hard to remember what she looked like before. She got it completely right by choosing a style that enhanced the elfin shape of her face. She also chose a style within the range of her natural hair type. Fine hair is not at its best-worn long, whereas heavy or naturally curly hair works well at shoulder length.

> **TIP** You can discover the shape of your face by drawing its outline in lipstick whilst you are holding a mirror at arm's length. Your shape will be revealed, clear as day – round, oval, long, heart-shaped, square.

Hairstyles that flatter your face:

- A long face can be shortened with a fringe and a chin-length cut with volume at the bottom.

- A square face is softened with curves and asymmetry.

- A heart-shaped face will look less so if the body of the hair is concentrated at chin level. Avoid extra height.

- If your jaw is long and sloping, like Jerry Hall, you should never wear your hair very short as it exposes the jaw.

- If the distance between your ear lobe and chin is short and you've a sharp angle where the jaw turns, like Audrey Hepburn, you can wear your hair any length.

- A round face works best when the hair comes forward onto the face. A soft fringe can work well too.

- Consider the head-to-body ratio. A close crop on a small head with a long neck and wide shoulders will look out of balance.

If your hair is **fine and straight**, don't wear it past shoulder length. If your hair is **curly** and your face is round, don't cut it short or add layers around the face. If your hair is **thick & coarse** you have a wide choice of styles but it's the hardest to look after. Don't cut it too short, stick to a strong shape.

The search for a great hairdresser has long been an emotive issue for women. So few of them seem to deliver what you really want. The best way to find one is to see a haircut you admire and find out who created it? Don't be shy about approaching a stranger in the street and asking her who styles her hair. She'll be flattered.

Never have your hair cut the day before something important – get it done a week or two before, so that if something goes wrong you have a chance to sort it out.

When you're trying a hairdresser out for the first time, don't ask for anything too extreme. Test them out with a 'half-an-inch off' trim and blow-dry first to see if you're on the same wavelength.

After that, never be afraid to talk to your stylist, and not about your next holiday. Ask him/her what he/she really thinks about your hair. You want the truth. This isn't about feelings but the perfect hair cut. Take charge of the situation; you want a hairstyle that suits you, not the latest fashion cut. Ask lots of questions. Think of the entire salon as your team.

Taking a picture from a magazine is a good idea as long as you're realistic enough to realise that magazine shots are 'styled for camera' so it may have taken hours to create the effect. Work out whether the model's cut will suit your face shape, hairline, bone structure, neck length and hair texture.

> 'Sophie's hair is quite thick and has a bit of a natural wave. I shape it every month with longer layers on top which gives a lot of choices. I tend to cut it wispy around the ends so even if she simply ties it back in a ponytail, it contours her face.'
>
> **John Barrett, stylist to Sophie Dahl**

Sophie Dahl is famous for being a blonde, so John Barrett's primary concern is to keep her hair both blonde and in great condition – which can be hard because her hair is sometimes styled for shoots several times a day. Sophie has a high lift colour, but because it's well looked after she doesn't pay the penalty of it looking dull and dry.

> **TIP** Never change everything – cut, colour and style – in one go. You need time to grow into it, just like your clothes style. Subtle seasonal changes are more flattering than total re-designs.

Colour guidelines

Choosing the right hair colour makes your face come alive and choosing the wrong one drains it completely. Supermodel Linda Evangelista constantly changes the shades of her hair and is one of those rare women who looks incredible whatever colour she chooses. She can be ash blonde one day and auburn the next because her skin and eyes work with everything. Her pale ivory skin is the perfect skin to take any hair colour as it has no pink in it.

If you have pink skin choose neutral tones like ash blonde, brown or dark brown. Don't go near red or yellow blonde. It won't work. Yellow/sallow skins can take dark rich tones with blue notes, like burgundy or deep auburn which counter balances sallow complexions. If you're lucky enough to have olive skin with dark hair, don't change a thing.

If you're determined to do it take the following advice:

- Sit in front of an honest mirror in daylight without makeup and ask yourself if your hair colour really suits you.

- If the answer is 'no', or 'I really want a change' consider what hair colour would flatter your skin tone.

- Also consider hair texture. Thin hair works better with an overall colour which needs to be retouched every five weeks; thick hair suits highlights–lowlights.

- When choosing a colourist, remember that an expert who specialises in colour is better than a hairdresser/permer who also does colour.

- Have a consultation first. Take pictures and colour samples and be honest about your hair history, i.e. perms, previous colour etc.

- Check how much maintenance your new colour will need, how much it will cost and what the contingency plan is if you don't like the colour.

- Try on wigs and hairpieces. Forget the style, focus on the colour.

- Check out the hair of the salon's staff. It will be an indication of their abilities.

On condition

For photo sessions, hairstylists often find it easier to work with a model with unwashed hair because it doesn't flop and is more manageable to work with. But in real life, nothing beats shampooing your hair every day, according to Philip Kingsley, who has been a leading celebrity trichologist for 30 years:

'It's a myth that this makes dry hair dryer and oily hair worse by stimulating the oil glands. Hair does not need oil; it needs water and moisture. Clean hair always looks its best. If you've got a style you can't wash every day — change it.'

Busy models are always looking for new ways of keeping their hair in top condition to counteract the constant back-combing, frying under hot studio lights, straightening and tonging and even submitting to whole colour changes.

An intensive conditioner is the secret weapon of every supermodel. They don't contain the same ingredients as ordinary conditioners, but have a high proportion of moisturisers, emollients and vegetable protein, which are all able to penetrate the hair shaft and repair damage and weakness.

TIP Supermodels swear by these two products to restore shine to tired hair: Philip Kingsley Elasticiser (a pre-shampoo conditioner) and Phytologies's Phyto 7 Daily Moisturiser (a leave-in, non-greasy blend of natural goodies).

Using the right type of products, specifically formulated for your hair type, makes a significant difference to the finished look of your hair:

- Fine hair loves being washed and conditioned every day. Keep it clean, well-moisturised and protect it from heated styling and the sun. Use a volumiser spray, but only on the roots.

- Thick hair is so strong that it often resists styling, so needs firm-hold products. Serum is the answer – it makes hair easier to handle and gives it fantastic shine.

- Curly hair is normally dry and needs a moisturising shampoo and intensive conditioner. Applying serum to the hair when wet helps to control it. Leave-in conditioner moisturises and protects.

The secrets of shiny hair

- Always use a shampoo and conditioner appropriate to your hair type.

- Spend more on a decent shampoo. Supermarket brands can be harsh.

- Use lukewarm water when you shampoo your hair and finish with a cold rinse.

- Blot, don't rub when you towel-dry your hair as this makes curly hair frizzy and damages fine hair.

- Don't brush wet hair. Comb it with a wide-tooth comb.

- When you dry your hair, don't use the dryer too hot. Treat your hair as you would a chiffon scarf.

- Don't brush your hair at night. It exhausts it.

- To heighten the effect of conditioner, comb it through your hair, always starting from the ends upwards. Leave 30 seconds. Then rinse thoroughly in cold water.

- Use the right product at the right time. Styling Cream is applied to hair before using heating appliances; mousse is applied before blow drying for texture and volume; thickening lotions are used for styling and setting, and serums define curl and add moisture to dry ends.

- Use just one styling product at any one time. A combination of serum, mousse and hairspray will only make your hair look flat, stiff and dull.

TIP This is the best way to create loose, undressed curls. Modern curls are not about big hair, root lift or curls that look obviously done. For natural waves take the following steps:

- Spritz dry hair (clean or dirty) with a homemade mixture of two tablespoons of salt, one teaspoon of sugar and half a pint of water and dry with hands or hairdryer.

- Wrap hair sections around heated tongs, ensuring each section is wrapped out and under the tongs, rather than up and over them.

- Apply a styling clay for extra texture and separation, and use your fingers rather than a brush to style.

- Instantly volumise flat hair by giving it a 'side-to-centre' parting (run it diagonally from one side of the crown).

- Never ever contemplate a perm, however much your hairdresser tries to convince you. Think about the contrast of the new hair growth to the chemically treated permed hair. (I know about this. A well-meaning hairstylist thought he would give me a 'little body perm' a month before my wedding. Result: no existing photographs of wedding/many honeymoon unsmiling hat shots.)

- In summer protect your hair with sunscreen products and hats.

- For very dry, brittle and damaged hair, mix an overripe avocado with the yolk of an egg. After shampooing, apply this mixture and leave on the hair for 30 minutes. Then rinse.

- To lift dull hair, wash with a mild shampoo and use a conditioner. Rinse out the conditioner and give the hair a final rinse using half-an-ounce of pure vinegar added to one pint of cold water.

TIP If you can't stand the smell of hairsprays, try using John Frieda's Thickening Lotion as you would a hairspray. It smells fantastic, and the hold is as natural and effective as favourites like Elnett.

To save time choose a hairstylist at a salon where you can have all your treatments done under one roof. American women call it 'multi-tasking'. When Jerry Hall has her colour done by Josh Wood (who also treats Elle Macpherson's locks) at Real Hair on Chelsea Green in London, she also has a manicure, pedicure and a trim.

5

How supermodels stay looking young

Is it a sad process for a beautiful model to age? Is she relieved to leave the centre stage and develop areas which don't focus on her looks? Or does she consider her beauty a 'gift' to be nurtured for the rest of her life?

Three ways to age

First, go with the flow. Learn to love your wrinkles which have given you some well-earned character in your face. Proudly tell people that you've earned your lines and a face-lift won't ever give your life a purpose.

Jean Shrimpton, the ultimate sixties supermodel happily follows this strategy. She always felt her beauty stopped her from developing her personality to the full. Jean was never comfortable in her role as the most famous model in the world, and it came as a welcome relief to her to put all the glamour behind her and retire to Cornwall, where, for many years, she ran a small hotel with her husband.

Second, wait until the damage of gravity, time and the sun start to show and then have on-going radical surgery and acquire a boyfriend half your age in an endless pursuit of youth.

This option has many followers in the acting profession in Hollywood, but in general is not a good idea. A narcissistic pre-occupation with self-perfection can easily develop, and it all becomes joyless and obsessive.

Third, take the subtle route and halt the obvious sign of ageing through a combination of cosmetic/medical/surgical regimes of prevention and repair.

This is the strategy followed, by many professional famous beauties, starting in their mid-thirties. They learn to adjust to the subtle changes the years etch onto their faces and bodies whilst aiming to look virtually the same throughout their adult life. Goldie Hawn is a good example of this regime. She hasn't noticeably changed, but admits to gently 'cheating'.

'I haven't had plastic surgery and I would never have it. I hate Botox because I think it makes people's faces look half-frozen, which is hopeless for my future as an actress.'
Jerry Hall

How to look younger than you are with make-up

Many women after 40 use the same make-up they did in their twenties and thirties, but the skin pales with age and changes in texture. Some women try to counter this by using sunbeds or trying darker foundations, but these tricks don't work. Skin needs to look fresh and radiant, not browner.

New cosmetics are very advanced and take into account the changes that occur when skin ages. There are now clever, imaginative formulas available that make the skin look younger and fresher, creating the illusion that you are ten years younger than you are.

The best are the 'skin illuminators', shimmery pink or peach fluids which add a youthful glow no amount of foundation can create. Undetectable to the eye, illuminators create the illusion of glowing skin.

Tricks for looking younger

- Always apply foundation in thin layers, little-by-little, rather than one thick unnatural layer.

- Always blend foundation over the eyelids as a primer for eyeshadow.

- Never apply a thick layer of concealer under the eye.

- Never use bright eyeshadow colours.

- Always stick to neutral-coloured eyeshadows in brown and grey.

- Never use eyeliner anywhere but the upper outer corners.

- Never wear dark lipstick colours. It makes them look thin and dull.

- Never wear a matte-textured lipstick. It makes them look dry/old.

- Always wear a palish, shimmery lipstick to make lips look fuller.

- Always use pink blusher, rather than peach, on apples of cheeks.

- Always avoid heavy powder, concealer, foundation round the eyes; it emphasises lines.

- Never use a matte eyeshadow, choose a slight shimmer.

The 'miracle' creams

More rubbish is spoken about anti-ageing creams than any other form of cosmetic treatment, and most of the bilge comes from the cosmetic companies themselves.

Currently these creams contain antioxidant vitamins (said to combat the effects of damage on the skin) and AHAs or fruit acids which are derived from chemicals found in milk and fruit. Ready to be launched soon as a 'revolutionary' new discovery are plant hormones like wild yam and soy in anti-ageing creams.

The claims to 'remove wrinkles and fine lines' are simply

untrue. These creams do not work, no matter how hi-tech they claim to be. The best they can do is to help diminish the appearance of fine lines on a superficial level.

In other words they plump up the skin for as long as you're wearing the product, and that's where it ends. They do no long-term good whatsoever beyond moisturising the top layer of skin and possibly getting rid of dead skin cells. Unless creams contain active ingredients, the sort only a doctor can prescribe, then that's all they will do.

To make serious inroads in delaying the skin-ageing process you have to:

- have decongesting facials and mild chemical peels;

- use medically prescribed lotions;

- eat properly;

- never smoke again;

- drink two litres of water a day;

- don't sunbathe;

- have regular Botox injections and plump your face with fillers.

Cheating it

At around 35, your skin becomes less hydrated, shows signs of environmental damage and begins to sag, as the tissue that binds collagen to the skin starts to break away.

Famous beautiful faces, contrary to what they would have the world believe, simply don't stay taut by magic.

Their owners have discreet non-surgical and sometimes minor surgical 'help'.

There are many new barely invasive procedures performed with little more than a mild anaesthetic, and hardly viewed any differently to having a leg wax or a facial. But many aspects of these procedures need to be addressed before rushing into them. How permanent are they? What are the long term risks? Is the person administering them truly qualified?

The true experts in age-maintenance, the top cosmetic surgeons, use a *smorgasbord* approach to the face – a bit of filling here, a bit of sandblasting there. They know that fillers can't help with sagging and bagging – only full surgery can do that.

Professor John Celin, one of the most popular cosmetic surgeons, says no amount of cream or injected collagen can achieve the instant results like Botox.

On lines that are the result of a loss of elasticity he injects a filler containing a hyaluric acid (Perlane is the current celebrity choice), which lasts about nine months, doesn't require an allergy test and is biodegradable.

Seriously cheating it

Cosmetic surgery is a scary thing to contemplate and should never be undertaken lightly. The effects are permanent, and if the surgeon you choose is over-enthusiastic, your face can lose its character forever.

Beauties who venture down this path choose their surgeon with great care, and never ever find him from an advert at the back of a magazine. Each surgeon has his acknowledged area of expertise and it's difficult to keep up with who is currently the best at what, unless you happen to be best friends with Cher.

Wendy Lewis is a well-respected adviser on cosmetic surgery, whose trademark is her independent and discreet advice. She has helped a number of professional beauties to choose the right surgeon for the job (see Resources, page 189).

My advice is to stop thinking about winning the 'Best Skin At Eighty' competition and have some fun in life. Better to have an interesting, laughing face, than a miserable flawless one.

I am, however, considering the fat recycling operation which transfers fat from my rump to my lips – so that I can finally agree with friends who tell me I'm always talking through my backside!

Molars, choppers and gnashers

For my money, a smile-lift is the best thing to knock ten years off your age. 'Power whitening' of teeth is a simple non-invasive and virtually fail-safe procedure in which the teeth are professionally bleached.

A bleaching gel is painted on to your teeth and a special activating light is placed over your mouth and the whitening begins. It takes an hour and can be performed every six months, although the results can last up to three years, depending on your red wine and cigarette intake. The results, though not cheap, are well worth the investment when you consider that 70% of people notice your teeth before anything else.

There's been heaps of hype about whitening toothpastes, but beware of them. Some whiteners harm the enamel by physically rubbing away the discoloration. Consumer magazine tests have proved these toothpastes have little or no effect, although the Dental Journal study found that Macleans Whitening Toothpaste was effective on many patients and say it is useful for an everyday toothpaste and whitener.

TIP Cut a strawberry in half and rub the juicy sides along your teeth to brighten and help remove stains.

On the shape of teeth, there's been a recent shift away from the perfect American smile to allow a bit of character. Kate Moss wouldn't be half as interesting without her pointy teeth, and Madonna's gap between her top front teeth is her trademark.

When I first arrived in New York to model, my agent was horrified by my Madonna-type gap and insisted I had it permanently 'fixed' before I started working. The fabulous model Lauren Hutton came to my rescue (she had a mega gap too) and gave me a small porcelain gadget to slip on for photo sessions to disguise the space.

We both like our gaps and didn't want them 'perfectionised', not least because they gave us impressive whistles with which we could hail cabs from five blocks away, making us the envy of rush hour Manhattan.

Part Two
Body

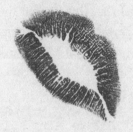

Models don't exactly come in all shapes and sizes but the shapes of their bodies differ more than you might imagine. They all have height, but some, like Twiggy and Kate Moss aren't as tall as you'd think – their proportions make them look tall.

Cindy Crawford and Elle Macpherson are so voluptuous they could have been Playboy bunnies, and others like Eric O'Connor and Stella Tennant are convincingly androgynous. This variety of shape means fashion designers and advertisers are able to choose the type of girl who best enhances their clothes and products.

Photographers also have their favourites, who are not necessarily similar to each other in shape. Rankin, one of the most innovative fashion photographers, loves working with Kate Moss and Helena Christensen. Both models are very different types – Kate is the 'waif' and Helena has a magnificent, statuesque body that could launch a thousand ships.

Though Helena's body is the one many other models say they would choose to have, those who become supermodels make it to the top by maintaining their natural body shape. They would not make themselves unnaturally thin in a misguided belief that this is what the fashion industry demands because they are happy in their own skins.

6

How models keep their bodies the right weight without dieting

There are many competent diet books and regimes, but none of them are suitable for models. The only thing that works for them is a sensible, long-term eating plan that enables them to maintain an even weight for the duration of their modelling career and beyond.

The stop/start effects of continuous dieting would be a nightmare for a girl who is booked for her consistent standard dress size. It's a fact that 95% of the weight lost in diets is regained at a later date.

Most reputable model agents will spot a girl who is struggling to be the correct weight for modelling. If they think she may have major problems maintaining her weight, they'll gently tell her that modelling is not the right career choice for her. Believe me, they have her best interests at heart. It does no good to force a body against its natural weight inclination. Not everyone is meant to be whippet thin – thank goodness.

> *The photographer Richard Avedon once told me, "Cindy you don't look good when you're thin, your face gets too skinny". So I used that as an excuse to be the weight that suits me rather than what was fashionable.'* Cindy Crawford

Model agents are also on the look-out for girls who have 'emotional' problems with food. Eating food should be a delicious experience, not something to beat ourselves up about. Permanently thinking about what can and can't be eaten perpetuates the focus on food. The constant fearing and counting of calories; obsessing about combining some foods and not others; having imagined wheat/dairy intolerances or always leaping on the scales have no place in a busy supermodel's life.

TIP A successful model realises that the only way to maintain her slim figure is by eating an amount of food in direct relation to what her body can burn off. Absolutely nothing else works.

She fuels her body for the job in hand. If she's been reading a book for three hours, she knows she's less likely to need a large three-course meal than if she's played three sets of tennis. She eats because she's hungry and stops when that hunger is satisfied.

The successful model eats sensibly and knows that to stay fit she needs foods from every category. She doesn't ban any foods from her plate. She simply eats less of what she knows puts on weight – fats, carbohydrates and sugar. It's not rocket science to work out that a pizza's going to make her fatter than a salad. She eats three meals a day because she knows this is the proven way to avoid the desire for snacks and because it keeps her energy levels well balanced.

Just because we're lucky enough to live in a country with bountiful supplies of food, doesn't mean we have to eat it all. Huge numbers of people in affluent societies eat vastly more than they need, through mindless, deliberate or unconscious over-eating causing many health problems known to be directly related to obesity.

Conversely, there are those who don't eat, punishing their bodies nutritionally for their emotional void. The inhabitants of poor countries never have eating disorders like bulimia and anorexia because they are too busy trying to find enough food to keep them alive.

If you seriously don't know whether you are under or overweight, do the Body Mass Index (BMI) test, which the medical industry use as a gauge. The BMI was devised a number of years ago by the US insurance industry, which linked weight to life expectancy, and this is the result of dividing your weight (in kg) by the square of your height (in metres).

BMI Formula

Weight (in kg) / Height^2 (in m^2)

E.G.

100 kg / (2^2) = 25

A normal BMI is between 20 and 25. Check yours:

BMI	Health Status
under 20	underweight
20–25	normal
25–30	overweight
30–35	obese
over 35	seriously obese

Sixteen ways to eat well and never diet

1. Eat real food (and restrict or ban processed/fake/junk food). Real food is anything that can be picked, gathered, milked, hunted or fished – food that is close to its natural origin.

2. Eats lots of chicken. It's a lean source of tryprophan, an essential amino acid that encourages the brain to produce serotonin, a 'happiness hormone'.

3. Don't ever skip meals. If your body goes for a long time without food, your blood sugar will drop, increasing your desire for sweet foods, making you more likely to snack.

4. Eat four times more vegetables and salad to protein (meat, fish, eggs, cheese) or carbohydrate (rice, pulses, bread, potatoes).

5. Never eat a meal that is larger than you can hold in your two cupped hands.

6. Eat five portions of fruit/vegetables every day – fresh, frozen or dried. This is not as hard as it looks. A glass of juice for breakfast, a large bowl of salad for lunch followed by a piece of fruit and two vegetables with your evening meal.

> **TIP** Live yoghurt is one of the legendary health foods of all time but not all brands have the beneficial culture *lactobacillus acidophilus*. Read the label carefully. Higher-fat yoghurts tend to have more calories and less calcium.

7. Don't forbid yourself any foods you desire. Human nature will make you want it more. Simply make allowances for it in your daily intake.

8. If you eat what feels good and nourishing, it will make you feel fulfilled and less likely to finish off with a chocolate brownie.

9. Try not to eat red meat more than three times a week. It can create a residue of toxins. Eat more fish instead.

10. Eat more nuts and seeds and fewer cakes and biscuits.

11. Eat lots of stir-fries, using stock, or a combination of soy sauce and white wine, instead of oil. Throw in heaps of garlic and ginger. They are both incredibly purifying.

12. Eat less butter, cream and cheese and switch to olive oil.

13. In a restaurant, order another starter instead of a main course. It will leave you room for a pudding without feeling guilty.

> **TIP** A cantaloupe melon, with its succulent orange-coloured flesh, cut in half and eaten with a spoon, is a filling, super-satisfying dessert. When buying a melon, choose a clean, unblemished one that feels heavy for its size.

14. If you eat more whole-grain carbohydrate food you will automatically reduce your intake of fat.

15. Choose sorbet or fresh fruit salad for pudding instead of ice cream.

16. If you want something, have it. Just eat less of it.

The model turned actress Jacqueline Bisset used a curious method to look older in a film she starred in recently, where she had to appear puffy and bloated in some scenes. She amazed make-up artists by literally ageing in front of them, simply by changing her diet.

By eating processed and junk food; takeaway Indian or Chinese food – or anything with too much salt – she found she could change her physique completely and look five or six years older in two days.

Ah, you may say, I don't eat muck like that; I eat freshly made food and when I don't have the time to cook I eat 'freshly prepared' meals from my favourite supermarket. Next time you buy one of these meals, run your eye down the contents on the pack and you will see how generously enhanced it is with artificial flavourings, colours, additives and E numbers.

The result of eating these meals regularly is a flabby body, fat around the middle, and accelerated ageing. That's all very well, you may say, but I simply don't have the time to cook every night.

Eating at home

At my deli in London we make a delicious one-pot meal in a huge pan. This can be a spring lamb casserole using new baby vegetables; chilli con carne using lean beef with lots of beans and chick peas, or anything that is nourishing and filling without being fattening. The contents of the huge pan are cooled, decanted into foil 'takeaway' containers and frozen.

We sell hundreds of these meals every week, because they're the healthy, modern answer to today's essential fast food. The beauty of a one-pot meal is that all the vitamins and minerals are retained in the sauce, they are easy to make and taste terrific. They contain no additives whatsoever, and quick-frozen food loses none of its nutrients through the freezing process.

One cooking session, making four different dishes, each with recipes for eight people, will give you enough meals to freeze for a month. No more supermarket shopping midweek; simply choose from one of your own 'prepared' meals each evening. Heat up the foil container in the oven for 45 minutes and open the wine. A complete meal with no fuss, no nasty E numbers and no washing up. No room in your freezer? Buy a bigger one with the money you save on 'freshly-prepared' meals at the supermarket.

'I'm the biggest cheese eater on the planet. My favourite shop in the world is a French cheese shop in Paris. I also adore pasta. I'm a big lover of food and I really enjoy that whole thing of eating and drinking with friends. But I guess I don't eat too much of these because I don't put on weight. Moderation is the key. Eat enough of your favourite foods to enjoy the delicious taste, but don't overdo it.' **Helena Christensen**

Never tempt fate when eating at home. Keep all the food in the kitchen. Having bowls of sweets and packets of biscuits in the living room or bedroom only increases temptation. Whatever you find the most difficult to resist – crisps, chocolate, fizzy drinks – keep out of the house.

Supermodel stir-fries

These recipes are unique because they're stir-fried quickly in water with added stock. The clean, delicious flavour of the food comes to the fore and guarantees you will never hanker after the greasy taste usually associated with stir-fried-in-oil food ever again.

The recipes work because they taste delicious, are sensationally good for you (they're all low fat and contain purifying garlic and ginger) – and are easy to prepare. Serve them with brown rice. All recipes serve 4–6.

Chicken and mange tout (snow peas)

400 g chicken breasts, cut into strips

150 g mange tout, trimmed

For the marinade

1 tablespoon ginger, finely chopped

3 cloves of garlic, chopped

1 tablespoon low salt soy sauce

2 tablespoons dry sherry

1 teaspoon cornflour

3 tablespoons chicken stock

freshly ground black pepper

For the sauce

4 tablespoons chicken stock

2 teaspoons cornflour

1 tablespoon dry sherry

METHOD

- Place the chicken in marinade for 15 minutes.

- Remove stems from the mange tout and blanche in boiling water for one minute and drain in colander.

- Drain chicken from marinade.

- Place the marinade in heated wok or large frying pan. Add the chicken and stir-fry for three minutes. Add mange tout and stir for one minute.

- Make the sauce by mixing the cornflour with the remaining ingredients. Add to the chicken and mange tout. Simmer and stir continuously for two minutes until sauce thickens. Serve immediately.

Fish with Cucumber

1 medium sized cucumber
3 tablespoons chicken or vegetable stock
1 clove garlic, chopped
1 teaspoon ginger, finely chopped
400 g white fish fillets, cut into thick slices
1 tablespoon dry sherry
2 shallots, diced
2 teaspoons low salt soy sauce
freshly ground black pepper to taste
2 teaspoons cornflour mixed with 1 tablespoon cold water

METHOD

- Slice the cucumber into thin discs and put to one side. Don't peel the cucumber.

- Bring the stock to the boil in a hot wok or non-stick frying pan and stir-fry the garlic and ginger for one minute.

- Reduce the heat, and add fish, sherry, shallots, soy sauce and pepper. Stir in the cornflour, mix and simmer for one minute.

- Add the cucumber slices, heat through and serve immediately.

Szechuan Chilli Beef

400 g beef fillet, cut into strips
1 clove garlic, finely chopped
1 onion, roughly chopped
1 teaspoon fresh ginger, finely chopped
2 fresh chillies, finely chopped
375 ml vegetable stock
1 tablespoon cornflour
1 tablespoon low salt soy sauce
freshly ground black pepper to taste
400 g Chinese cabbage, shredded

METHOD

- Stir-fry beef, garlic, onion, ginger and chillies over high heat in stock until tender – about two minutes.

- Mix cornflour with soy sauce. Simmer and stir continuously until sauce thickens, about two minutes.

- Season with ground black pepper.

- Place shredded Chinese cabbage on top and stir-fry for two minutes.

Prawns with Mange Tout

16 mange tout, trimmed
3 tablespoons chicken stock
1 teaspoon fresh ginger, finely chopped
1 clove garlic, chopped
1 fresh red chilli, chopped
300 g fresh uncooked prawns, shelled and de-veined
freshly ground black pepper
2 teaspoons cornflour mixed with 1 tablespoon cold water
2 tablespoons dry sherry

METHOD

- Blanche mange tout in boiling water for one minute and set aside.

- Bring the stock to the boil in a hot wok or non-stick frying pan and stir-fry ginger, garlic and chilli for one minute.

- Add prawns and pepper. Stir-fry for four minutes.

- Add cornflour mix and sherry and simmer for one minute.

- Add mange tout, heat through and serve.

Brown rice

Brown rice is packed with B vitamins and fibre. It can be broken down and digested quickly and its great absorption soaks up toxins in the gut.

ABSORPTION METHOD

This method ensures perfectly cooked rice every time (1 cup of rice to 2 cups of water):

- Wash the rice in cold water and drain in a colander.

- Bring the rice and water to the boil in a large saucepan.

- Turn heat to very low. Cover saucepan with tight fitting lid and cook for 35–40 minutes. Don't lift the lid during this time.

- Remove from the heat, uncover and fluff rice with a fork.

Eating out

If you're lucky enough to eat out regularly the key is to choose what you're eating rather than letting it choose you. Always think carefully before you order. Eating Italian food doesn't always have to be starchy pasta or pizza – try an antipasto platter or meat and vegetables. If you really can't resist that burger, ditch half the bun and eat it as an open sandwich.

The best way to resist unhealthy food is to stop and analyse its provenance, e.g. how far it has travelled from its origins. Just imagine what ingredients go into a hot dog. A cold dog, perhaps. It literally defies description. The further that food has been processed from its natural state, the more unhealthy it is for the body.

'I eat reasonably sensibly because I was brought up to eat well. I have lots of vegetables when I eat at home. I like fish but don't cook it for myself. The most important part of my diet is potatoes. I love them and eat them every day.

Also cereals for high fibre. Sometimes I eat a few sweets when I feel like it but it's not a big deal.'
Catherine Hurley

The next time you order a rich sherry trifle or a French meat dish drenched in foie gras and three cream sauces ask yourself, what is this? How far is this from fresh, real food? When you gaze upon a huge piece of runny, unpasteurised Brie and want to scoff the lot, see it as a large helping of fat sitting in your intestines for three days. Ditto a cold bacon sandwich, or a large bar of Toblerone.

> **TIP** When you don't have reliable scales, keep a pair of old jeans that fit you perfectly at hand. If you suspect you've added a few pounds, try on the jeans and if they're tighter than usual – you have.

You truly are what you eat. When you swallow food, it doesn't just go away somewhere and hide. It becomes a part of your body. That's why the tactile pleasure of eating a fresh mango usurps the dubious delights of downing a doughnut.

Don't give yourself excuses to eat bad food. If you find yourself in a mediocre restaurant or hotel, simply take a tip from the supermodels. In this situation they will only order food that has to be cooked on the spot, and therefore is totally fresh, like an omelette, or grilled meat and a salad you dress yourself.

Travel

Airline food is usually of poor quality and models, who travel constantly, know to ring the airline ahead and order the vegetarian menu, which is always fresher and purer than the bog-standard offerings. On short haul trips models pack their own goody bags – unsalted freeze-dried nuts, a banana or apple, a couple of hard-boiled eggs and the ubiquitous bottle of mineral water.

Kicking the sugar habit

Deep-fried starters, leftovers and pizza may be easier to divorce than chocolate. The sugar hit is a seductive beast even though we know it makes us fat, spotty, have bad teeth and plays havoc with our energy levels. When we eat chocolate, we have an instant energy boost; feel tired; then reach for another sugar fix – a cycle that can be literally nausea-inducing. Eating too much chocolate controls our moods, gives us headaches and migraines and ruins our skin – but still we love it.

There are two options for the chocolate addict: reduce your sugar intake gradually, or go cold turkey and banish sugary foods completely. The first strategy probably works best long-term.

Cutting out sugary foods for a week or so will make you feel sufficiently in control of your sweet tooth to eat the occasional sweet treat. Combine this with cutting out coffee, tea, fizzy drinks and sports and energy drinks. The caffeine they contain can disrupt your new energy levels, the initial buzz often being followed by a low that can trigger a craving for something sweet.

Quash sugar cravings with chromium-rich foods like shellfish, cheese, baked beans and wholemeal products such as wholemeal bread, cereals and pastas. Protein-packed foods such as chicken, fish, eggs, pulses, lentils and lean red meat also ward off sugar urges.

If you eat more whole-grain foods, along with plenty of vegetables and fresh fruits (although the fruit will give you sweetness, their fibre content will suppress any further sugar cravings) your blood-sugar level will remain more constant.

> **TIP** Carry a small bottle of vanilla essence in your handbag and take a sniff of it or rub it on the back of your hand every time you feel a sugar craving coming on. It really works.

Reward your body for staying clear of unhealthy foods by spoiling it in other ways.

Let your body know how much you appreciate its support, rather than always criticising it for not being the perfect shape. Your body is a complete miracle, it works hard to keep you fit and shouldn't be ignored or treated with anything less than total respect.

Ten treats your body will love on a regular basis:

1. Being massaged.

2. Lounging in front of an open fire.

3. Swimming naked.

4. Being moisturised from head to toe.

5. Eating fresh mango.

6. Lying in a field of long grass.

7. Watching a good film.

8. Walking down a country lane.

9. Reading a great book.

10. Drinking a superb glass of wine.

7

Finding the perfect exercise that becomes a pleasure for life

Sticking with exercise has as much to do with your head as your body. If you follow the wrong workout regime for you it becomes boring and if you overdo it when you start, it won't last long. Two thirds of people leave health clubs and gyms within the first six months of joining. The key to maintaining a fit body is finding an enjoyable exercise regime that is absolutely right for you – and keeping it up.

You will never stay with a fitness regime long-term if it makes you feel bored, guilty, pressurised, over-competitive or resentful. Choosing the right regime in the first place is crucial and joining a gym is not the only option. If you like time to yourself, try cycling or brisk walking. If you lack confidence, take up one of the martial arts, and if you feel you need a tough regime, copy Sophie Dahl and adopt a personal trainer.

If you're seriously contemplating a Sophie Dahl type transformation, then a truly dedicated and focused fitness programme is essential. With the help of her personal trainer, Dave Bennett, Sophie totally changed the shape of her body with a ninety minute fitness routine three times a week for three years, dropping three dress sizes and losing more than five inches from her waist in just six weeks.

Going for it?

But if you've joined a gym because you feel a bit guilty from eating too much Christmas food, you probably won't go back after the first few visits and will join the thousands of people a year, like me, whose membership cards gather dust.

That's because your subconscious mind doesn't think of the exercise you have chosen as fun and a positive experience, so it sabotages your conscious attempts to get to the gym, making it very difficult to motivate yourself.

If you have a job where you dash around and use heaps of energy, you obviously need less exercise than if you sit in an office all day. And if your idea of fun is clubbing and dancing in the evening, you need less exercise than if your hobby is going to the movies.

> *'Losing weight is not about the things you should not do; it's about the things you should do. You can stay slim without starving yourself, and don't need expensive gyms or exercise equipment to keep fit.'* **Jerry Hall**

The other thing to consider about gyms is that the people who do regular high-intensity sessions there, tend to reward themselves in-between sessions by eating more food. They think they're burning off far more calories in a gym session than they actually are.

Even if you do 45 minutes in an exercise class or on equipment, such as a treadmill or a bicycle, you're unlikely to work off more than 300 calories. Gym sessions should be the icing on the cake rather than the only activity you ever do.

Pushing it

Exercise regimes go in and out of fashion and it is important not to get caught up in a regime because it's fashionable rather than what suits your lifestyle. Your body desires maintenance not violent punishment.

The Jane Fonda 'high impact' aerobics of the eighties involved constant pounding of the joints and going for the 'burn' and this has proved to be bad news for the body long-term, often destroying cartilage that protects the joints and putting even 30 year olds at serious risk of osteoarthritis.

If it's important for you to gain and retain a stomach like a washboard, then there are benefits to be gained from a formal or structured programme, which includes cardiovascular work and weights. This kind of exercising vigorously improves your stamina, conditions your heart and lungs, increases your flexibility and tones and strengthens your muscles – as well as giving you energy.

Stretching it

If you want to lengthen and tone muscles and look leaner without building up muscle, then yoga or Pilates is the answer. They use specific breathing patterns and involve intense, deep stretching regimes that produce a long lean body without any bulking of the muscles. Pilates is a gentler, safe alternative to yoga without the spiritual emphasis.

Supermodel Christy Turlington is an avid yoga devotee and embraces its spirituality. She believes that yoga helps you get in touch with who you are, and what you want, and helps to make your ideas become realities.

Iyengar yoga is a good option for beginners as it puts great emphasis on correct postures. Sivananda yoga and Viniyoga are also gentle, but never be tempted to try Ashtanga yoga (as close as aerobics as yoga gets) unless your body is used to high octane exercise. This is 'power yoga' and needs a tough discipline, although devotees say it is the best workout ever.

> **TIP** Choose an exercise where you're able to chat easily – without puffing and panting – whilst you're doing it. If you feel strained, it's too much for you.

Loving it

Several top models use mini trampolines. I'm currently mad about trampolines and want one for my birthday. I can't think of any other form of exercise that's as much fun whilst doing you so much good. Well maybe one.

Especially beneficial for thighs, trampolining is the ultimate exercise for tackling cellulite because rebounding strengthens the ligaments and tones all the major muscles and connective tissue.

Other types of cardiovascular exercise like dancing, swimming, cycling , jogging, golf, tennis and brisk walking are also good for strengthening the heart and lungs, improving circulation and excellent for burning calories and body fat.

The Quatar exercise bike (currently only available in America) is another model favourite with girls based in New York. It has a screen attached with visuals of different countries – so you can cycle through Calcutta and end up in Paris. Not bad for a morning's workout.

Doing it

Consistency is the important thing and when a model finds herself on location, or away from her normal exercise regime, she makes the best of what's available. Running up and down hotel stairwells; doing sit-ups in her bedroom; discovering the nearest available swimming pool and walking round the nearest park are all beneficial alternative regimes which clear the head and keep the body trim.

> *'Everyday when I'm at home, I take my baby in his stroller for two or three hours — not power walking, I'll stop here and there — but it makes a difference, at least I'm out there.'*
>
> **Helena Christensen**

One of the most under-rated but a good-all-round exercises is fast walking. It's a great antidote to depression, keeps you alert and manages to exercise every part of you. These days it's my exercise of choice. I take my dog for a thirty minute brisk walk each morning and every evening. My motivation is the mutual pleasure we both gain from the experience, and the routine has become as familiar as brushing my teeth.

Six simple ways to stay fit:

1. Walk everywhere a little bit faster.

2. Stand rather than sit whenever possible; stand up to take and make a phone call; deliver messages to colleagues rather than e-mailing them.

3. Hide all the remote controls and change television/stereo channels manually. This could burn off 300–400 calories a week.

4. Always use the stairs rather than a lift or escalator.

5. Walk as much as possible throughout the day (park in the

furthest space away from the supermarket or office door, get off at an earlier bus stop than usual).

6. Try to find time in the week for proper exercise such as swimming or going to the gym, but see it as the icing on the cake, not your only form of activity.

The well-being hit list:

- Don't get too thin. Subcutaneous fat helps to plump out wrinkles and cheeks and keeps skin looking healthy.

- Don't run. Constant pounding motion causes the skin to lift and droop, resulting in elastic tissue losing its natural twang.

- Protect your skin from the sun. As if you didn't know!

- Get lots of sleep. Skin repairs itself at night when it's not busy defending itself against sunlight, pollution and other environmental invasions...the best skin repair time is between 11 p.m. and 3 a.m.

- Protect skin cells internally. Take vitamin C and eat food rich in nutrients that help protect the skin – avocados, berries, citrus fruits, grapes, spinach, broccoli and carrots.

- Accept your natural shape. Adjust your intake of food to suit your metabolism. Staying within an acceptable weight and increasing exercise makes you feel younger and more energetic.

- Minimise stress. By breathing deeply and counting each breath up to ten. If your mind wanders, start again.

Eventually you will be able to 'quieten your mind' without counting.

■ Laugh. Listen to a comedy CD on the way to work. Buy a joke book and memorise a joke a day. If you can't do anything about it, don't worry about it.

■ Don't yo-yo diet. The more the skin has to stretch and contract, the more it loses its elasticity.

■ Take up yoga/Pilates. Two forms of exercise that elongate the muscles and make the body leaner.

8

Know your body treatments

As life gets more stressful, 'feel-good' body treatments are becoming more and more popular. Spas are springing up everywhere and hotels and health resorts no longer boast about their fabulous beaches, but of their lavish pampering facilities.

What's out there? The A–Z of alternative therapies

- Acupuncture. The ancient Chinese art of sticking very fine needles into precise points along the body's energy channels to treat disease and maintain health.

- Aromatherapy Massage. Using essential oils of plants and flowers.

- Ayurveda. Ancient Indian system of medicine designed to achieve a state of health through a blend of meditation, yoga, astrology, herbal medicine and dietary advice.

- Chiropractors. Work directly on joints to correct joint and muscle disorders by manipulating the supporting bones.

- Chinese Medicine. Used mainly for chronic skin conditions like eczema.

- Flower Remedies. Tinctures of flower essences used to improve the body and mind's energy levels and mood.

- Homeopathy. Uses a minute amount of substance, that in large quantities would make you ill, to cure a condition it would otherwise create.

'I try to get regular massages and I have acupuncture once a week, which I find strengthens my immune system, relaxes me and slows me down when things are hectic.'

Christy Turlington

- Hypnotherapy. Asking a hypnotist to share and influence your unconscious thoughts and fears.

- Kinesiology. A muscle-strength testing technique to identify imbalances in the body increasingly used to detect food intolerances and allergies

- Massage. Many types…see page 93.

- Naturopathy. A collage of natural therapies using what

nature provides (sleep, organic food, pure water, exercise etc) to help the body heal itself

- Neurolinguistic Programming. A Californian behavioural technique that aims to help you achieve your goals.

- Osteopathy. Working on the muscles and ligaments surrounding joints, often with manipulation. To correct muscle disorders.

- Pilates. Developed in New York in the 1930s, a series of controlled exercises that work the abdominal and back muscles.

'There's nothing like reflexology for me, it's the best. I find it so relaxing at the time and afterwards I feel as though I'm walking on air.'
Catherine Hurley

- Radionics. A paraphysical method of diagnosis and treatment utilising the faculty of extra-sensory perception.

- Reiki. Japanese technique for re-balancing the 'universal life energy' of a person via healing.

- Reflexology. Freeing energy and healing particular parts of the body that correspond to pressure points on the foot.

- Yoga. Spiritual and physical exercise programme that enhances well being.

Pampering ourselves is wonderfully indulgent and repairs and prepares us for the next onslaught of real life. There's nothing more therapeutic than a good massage, given by a true professional, rather than someone who's just completed the right number of weekend courses! And yoga and Pilates should be classified as a way of life rather than as alternative therapies.

It's harmless and enjoyable to try reflexology, aromatherapy and the rest and I strongly believe therapies like acupuncture, homeopathy, osteopathy and chiropractic manipulation have a real place in our lives and make a serious and lasting difference.

How to decide what's right for you

The area gets tricky when metaphysics comes into play and we are asked to put our faith in the person administering the treatment. Some of the practitioners of the more esoteric therapies appear to be foolish dreamers, as deluded as those they seek to delude.

There is no monitoring body for most types of alternative therapies, which means literally anyone can set up shop with no qualifications whatsoever, or at best a 'training course'. Becoming an 'alternative therapist' or councillor often appeals to people from troubled backgrounds, who are not always the best equipped to administer 'calm' to others, so do some major research before embarking on a course of treatment that sounds appealing.

There are other 'therapists' who are cleverer at disguising their assets, but who are obviously complete charlatans who charge the earth for their useless 'cures' because they see there's money in hope, and the more desperate the hope, the richer the pickings.

> **TIP** Don't always think the 'feel-good' factor is enough to justify the cost of a treatment. Everyone feels better after lying on a couch and being given total attention and hands-on gentle touching. Ask yourself how different you really feel.

Many therapists will tell you that several visits are needed in order for you to feel the benefits. If you want to give them the benefit of the doubt, try two or even three treatments. If it's not an open and shut case by then, I have only one thing to say – a fool and her money are easily parted.

On the few occasions I've been tempted to lie down and have people apply their various 'talents' to the improvement of my energy levels the only 'extraordinary feeling of lightness' I've ever had is in my wallet. Sometimes Chaka Khan when chakras can't.

However, there are good practitioners out there, and the model's favourite is Dr Mosaref Ali at the Integrated Medical Centre. Kate Moss swears by Dr Ali and with good reason. He successfully combines conventional and alternative medicine and his traditional therapies are based on his belief of seeing human beings as part of a whole – body, mind and spirit – and as part of nature. He teaches how to heal yourself and the importance of fresh air, rest, yoga-based exercise, organically produced food and massage.

No need to knead

A plain old Swedish massage is no longer the only option available. All sorts of new massage techniques are popping up everywhere, to stimulate or to relax, to stretch the mind as well as the body.

I believe that a good massage, given by an experienced and knowledgeable masseur is the most beneficial treatment you can have. You feel and see instant results. Massage improves your circulation, relieves knotted muscles, balances your mind and the hands-on touch of a good masseur is re-assuring and soothing. Treat yourself to something on the massage menu.

Twelve types of massage and their techniques

1. Aromatherapy. Uses fab-smelling essential oils to relax, revive or invigorate the body and mind.

2. Chinese. A light massage concentrates on acupressure points to stimulate the flow of energy around the body.

3. Deep Tissue. Deep work on neuro-muscular tissues to help tune body and mind.

4. Holistic. A massage which aims to soothe and ground the patient bodily, emotionally and physically.

5. Heller Work. Deep-tissue massage helps re-align the body and release tensions and pent-up emotions.

6. Indian Head Massage. Stimulates the muscles and the body's lymphatic system by working on the head.

> **TIP** Most body treatments work better if you're nude. If you feel uncomfortable without your knickers, your therapist won't mind if you keep them on. A good therapist will never judge a client's body, and will always use towels to cover nudity in areas they're not working on.

7. Manual Lymphatic Drainage. A gentle but powerful technique to improve lymphatic system flow and decongest water retention/bad diet

8. Shiatsu. Finger pressure applied along the body's meridians promotes harmonious energy flow/releases tension.

9. Sports. Basic, no-frills rub down focusing on loosening and lengthening muscles for optimum functioning.

10. Swedish. Traditionally uses talc rather than oil. Much kneading, pummelling of muscles, chopping movements across the back. Dated regime.

11. Ayurvedic. Assisted yoga stretching. Expands the mind as well as muscles. Lots of oil.

12. Thai. Yoga limb stretches, followed by foot massage – the masseur's feet not yours.

Vitamins and minerals — why not?

Recently, a model I know ended up in hospital for four days with a mystery illness. After various tests it transpired that she had been to a naturopath and was taking 700 times the recommended daily amount of magnesium for chronic fatigue. When she stopped taking the supplement, her condition cleared up immediately.

It amazes me that you can walk into a chemist or health food shop and buy toxic levels of vitamins and minerals and no one will stop you or guide you about dosage or the danger of combinations.

For example, certain supplements require other vitamins and minerals if they're going to do their job properly. If you take iron, you'll need to ensure you're getting enough vitamin C too, or the body won't absorb it. If the vitamins are water-soluble (like B & C) then at normal levels any excess is simply flushed out of the body. But the fat-soluble vitamins A, D and E are stored and can cause tissue and organ damage if too much is taken.

In certain cases, supplements are invaluable. Vitamin C is a great antioxidant and immunity booster, wonderful for internal skin repair. It hates being stored, so may have a higher nutrient value than fresh oranges on shelves, picked weeks ago, and ripened in transit with chemicals.

If you're going through a stressful time – your normal

healthy eating regime is disrupted and you 're drinking too much coffee and alcohol, smoking or in a smoky environment – your B vitamin and magnesium levels will be depleted and a daily, good quality (the cheap ones are useless) multi-vitamin pill makes sense. Vegetarians and pregnant women need added supplements but, in the main, I believe that if you are eating a healthy diet, and your life is normal, pouring vitamins into your system is unnecessary and a waste of money.

HANDLE WITH CARE

	Why Take It?	Harm if you overdo it
Vitamin A	■ Boosts immunity. ■ Combats skin disorders.	■ Excessive doses linked to cancer scares. ■ Harmful in early pregnancy.
Vitamin B6	■ Combats depression. ■ Combats PMT symptoms.	■ More than 500 ml a day causes nerve damage.
Vitamin C	■ Boosts immunity. ■ Antioxidant. ■ Repairs skin.	■ Diarrhoea and cramps.
Vitamin D	■ Helps promote strong bones and teeth.	■ Nausea. ■ Vomiting. ■ Headache. ■ Depression.
Vitamin E	■ Maintains healthy cells.	■ More than 1000 mg causes blood thinning.
St John's Wort	■ A herbal anti-depressant.	■ Can interfere with contraceptive pill.

	Why Take It?	Harm if you overdo it
Evening Primrose Oil	■ Skin and period problems.	■ Can provoke epileptic attacks in susceptible patients.
Iron	■ Cures anaemia.	■ Constipation. ■ Diarrhoea. ■ Possible death from heart or liver failure.

If you are taking any of these supplements, check and double check with your general practitioner that you are within the recommended dose and ensure that any other medication you may be taking does not conflict with these supplements and vitamins.

9

How models keep cellulite at bay

Everywhere you look there's conflicting information about the causes and treatments of cellulite. Because it's not recognised by the medical profession, there's no prescribed treatment, leaving the door open for all sorts of quackish 'cures' which don't have to be officially regulated.

Beauty salons only need to claim that a treatment works for it to be sold as such. Ingredients don't have to be listed on products and there are around 10,000 websites trying to sell a cure for cellulite.

With no official guidelines, the best advice appears to be the direct experience of the women who watch out for this problem more than most – the supermodels. Even they are not immune, as the tabloid press gleefully reminds us, but they do have access to the top treatments and information – for the most beneficial results – which I have collated, in this section.

What is it?

....

Even skinny young models get cellulite – subcutaneous fat caught in the webbing of fibrous tissue that connects the skin with deeper tissue layers. But it's a lifestyle thing, a reaction to modern living, rather than a 'fat' issue.

Cellulite is a reflection of the body's inability to process hormones and toxins effectively, combined with poor circulation, lack of exercise and a less than perfect diet. Chinese women don't have it because they eat a pure low-fat diet and have active lifestyles.

The reason women (men don't get it) become disillusioned about cellulite is because it's a high maintenance problem that must be tackled from many angles, both inside and out, to see any improvement. It's no good rubbing in some cream if you don't change your diet. **You must combine the right diet, massage and exercise to get results.**

Diet

....

The first step is to eliminate obvious toxins from your diet and stop 'beverage abuse' by cutting out coffee, tea, fizzy drinks (these drinks contain chemicals you shouldn't put down your drain, let alone your throat). Stop eating fatty foods and ones with additives. Reduce your intake of wheat and dairy foods and eat as many fresh whole-foods as possible. Stick with the classic healthy diet of five portions of fruit and vegetables a day, plenty of antioxidant rich cruciferous vegetables like broccoli, pak choi and cauliflower, and protein from fish and white meat.

It's impossible to eliminate all the toxins but a good daily intake of water will go a long way to helping. If you find two litres a day too much to drink, work out the correct, manageable quantity for your body by drinking one 8 fl oz glass of water per 20 lb of your body weight. And avoid smoking; it reduces the skin's elasticity, making the orange peel more visible.

TIP Bathing is a great way to expel toxins. Soak yourself in water softened with alkaline bath salts. Try to do this two or three times a week.

Exercise

Regular exercise is vital for cellulite busting, not only for reducing the body fat including cellulite, but also for toning the muscles under the fat, thus minimising the mottled effect. Traditional body-toning exercises like aerobics or weight training don't help cellulite. The best fat-burners are gentle, long-lasting activities like cycling and swimming. A mini trampoline is excellent, as rebounding is the best way to strengthen ligaments and tone muscles. Simply jumping up and down for ten, building up to thirty minutes a day, strengthens all the major muscle groups and connective tissue.

Skin-brushing

Dry skin-brushing plays a major part in shifting stubborn deposits of cellulite. It breaks up the fat and improves lymphatic drainage from the thighs. The trick is not to brush too hard. What you're trying to do is stimulate lymphatic drainage, not blood circulation, so if your skin starts to redden as you brush, you're going too hard and will only draw more toxins to the area. Call me sad, but skin brushing is my favourite thing in the whole world. Here's what you do:

- Buy a long-handled pure bristle brush designed for the job. (see Resources).

- Before your morning shower, brush your skin starting from the soles of your feet up along your legs to your buttocks.

- Brush in one direction only, in single upwards strokes towards the middle of your body, using firm but gentle pressure.

- After your legs, thighs and torso, front and back, brush both arms from the tips of the fingers to the tops of your shoulders and your scalp and neckkkkk…whoops I'm getting carried away.

- Finally brush your neck and the top of your chest downwards.

The effect of skin-brushing makes you feel very tingly and brilliantly light-headed and if you finish your shower with a cold rinse, you'll be buzzing for the rest of the day. If you do this two or three times a week, I promise you'll have clearer skin, brighter eyes and boosting your lymph means you'll have fewer colds, clearer sinuses and less puffiness. You mustn't skin brush however if you have an infection, cancer, high blood pressure or a heart condition.

Creams
....

No creams can dissolve cellulite. If they did that to the fat cells in the thighs, imagine what they would be doing to the rest of the body. Any cosmetic company that claims anything else is trying to sell-you-light. But, similar to face creams that instantly plump out lines (but wash off later) there are creams that appear to make the flesh look smoother, firmer and healthier, even though the underlying cellulite is still there.

Cellulite creams are expensive, often twice or three times as much as a moisturiser. But it is the direct contact between the user's hand massaging the creams on the troubled area, rather than the creams themselves that make a difference.

TIP Realise that cellulite creams work by tightening the surface skin. No commercial (non-prescribed) substances can penetrate the outer layer of skin unless it's broken or unhealthy.

Massage

After your bath or shower, firmly massage the cellulite areas with an oil, cream or gel.

Olive oil or body cream will be as good as any fancy creams. Massage helps disperse the toxins and stimulates sluggish fat cells. Always massage in circular motions with firm pressure towards the heart.

Okay that's the lot. I know it's a tall order but if you make a regular effort in every direction, two or three times a week, you will see your cellulite improve. Remember it is the combination of all the remedies that makes it work.

Anti-cellulite checklist:

- Avoid processed, rich food – eat fresh whole-foods instead.

- Do some vigorous exercise e.g. dancing, speed walking, cycling, swimming and trampolining.

- Skin brush. It's simple and makes you feel great.

- Drink plenty of water.

- Don't smoke.

- Massage the skin.

- Don't expect miraculous results too soon.

- Don't take cellulite too seriously. The most discerning women have it.

10

What supermodels really think about the sun

Despite all the adverse publicity about the obvious harmful effects of the sun on our skin, most of the supermodels I spoke to said they yearned for a gently golden body from time-to-time and that the sun made them feel happy and healthy. That they love the sun as much as they loathe its harmful effects is as true as the fact that a tanned body makes them look slimmer, healthier and better in summer clothes.

It's one thing to say, in the middle of winter, that you simply won't go near the sun next summer, but the fact is – the sun is seductive. It makes us feel good. How many people can honestly say they have never succumbed to having a gentle real tan?

I'm not endorsing lying in the sun for hours on end, but I am saying be realistic and be prepared to tan safely if the urge takes you, which means slowly, carefully and with the right sunscreen.

Although we're told that skin damage caused by ultraviolet rays is responsible for 80% of fine lines and wrinkles, we shouldn't be quite as scared of the sun as we are. In sensible doses it has enormous health benefits, helping us to produce the vitamin D we need for healthy bones and skin.

Elle Macpherson gets it completely right – a sun-kissed glisten that makes her look amazing. We're definitely not talking the mahogany leather look here. A mid to dark tan looks vulgar, hard and ageing. The aim is a delicious gentle summer glow like Elle's. There are simply two solutions.

How to achieve the perfect compromise

Short-term

Fake it with an instant tan. They've all dramatically improved and are now easy to apply and not so smelly and streaky. Formulas include mousse, gel, spray, lotion or liquid. St Tropez is still as popular as ever – salon or home applied. This is how to make it look real if you're bronzing at home:

- Do a patch test the night before to check out the shade.

- Make sure legs are hair-free to ensure smooth colour.

- Exfoliate body with loofah or body scrub, especially elbows, knees and heels. Apply body lotion to dry areas.

■ Thoroughly exfoliate face with facial scrub or wet muslin.

■ Never apply the tan directly onto problem areas: feet, ankles, knees, elbows and hands. Instead, put it on the thighs, shins, forearms and so on, massage it in, and then sweep a little product over the tricky areas.

■ To avoid the tanned-palm syndrome, rub a small amount of exfoliator between your hands before rinsing the palms carefully.

■ Sweep the back of the hands over a tanned area to top up any colour wiped off during rinsing.

■ Don't sit on sheets or fabric furniture or put on good clothes until the formula has sunk in, whatever the instructions say.

TIP If you accidentally get fake tan on your palms, apply whitening toothpaste and leave for several minutes – it removes all traces of stain.

Medium-/long-term tan

If you've decided to throw caution to the wind for a bit of colour, there are major precautions you must take. Everyone who goes in the sun needs sunscreen. The higher the number, the more protection a cream offers. Sun protection factor (SPF) numbers relate to the length of time you can stay in the sun without burning.

Fair skins can tolerate 10–15 minutes in full sun. Multiply that initial period of ten minutes by an SPF of 15 and it gives you 2½ hours' protection (150mins). That's your daily ration. Darker skins can take longer but need to apply sunscreen regularly. Avoid the sun between 11 a.m. and 3 p.m., when the sun's rays are at their strongest, and if you are in Australia, halve the times above and up the SPF.

- Never use sunbeds, pre-tan accelerators or tanning pills. They lower the skin's defence against UV rays.

- Build up your tan very slowly. It won't last long if you burn.

- Never lie out in the sun after 11 a.m. and before 3 p.m.

- On the first day apply a high factor sunscreen that protects you from wrinkle-forming UVA as well as the burning UVB. (Think of UVA as ageing, UVB as burning). Use factor 30 for the chest and face; 15 for the rest of the body. Apply 20 minutes before going out in the sun, so you don't sweat it off.

- Apply sunscreen liberally every one to two hours and immediately after swimming.

- Gradually reduce the factor, except on the face and chest.

- Make sure the entire eye area is lightly covered with an SPF 25 specially made for eyes and lips. Combined lip and eye sticks are easy to use.

- Make sure you have a hat with you to protect your face, neck and hair. Your hair won't protect your scalp from getting burnt.

- Keep applying fake tan to the face and chest so you won't be tempted to sunbathe unprotected.

- Wear sunglasses where possible. Exposure of the eye area to the sun contributes to decreasing vision as you get older.

- Exfoliate every evening to prevent peeling.

- Use a PABA-free sunscreen. PABA is short for para-aminobenzoic acid, and it can cause irritation to the skin and stain clothing.

- If your skin is dry, choose a cream; if it's oily, opt for a light-textured lotion or gel. Be generous with your sunscreen. Applying too thinly can reduce the SPF by half.

- Don't use anti-ageing products, especially fruit acids or retinal creams.

TIP When lying in the sand, prevent your thighs from horizontally spreading by nonchalantly hollowing out two leg-shaped furrows in the sand. Position your towel or sarong over the furrows, and place a leg in each furrow.

How to have the best body on the beach

....

Never wave to people unless your upper arm is taut and firm otherwise your arm won't stop waving.

Avoid a bloated stomach by substituting live yoghurt and cold soup for fruit and vegetables. Avoid diet food, especially diet yoghurt – they swell the stomach to give the impression of fullness. Avoid fizzy drinks, pasta, bread and beans. Don't chew gum or drink from a bottle or through a straw as it makes you swallow air.

Dry your skin thoroughly with a towel after swimming in the sea. Don't let the sun dry the water on your skin as it will leave a layer of salt behind which badly dries the skin.

Never sit up straight or your stomach will look like a stack of tyres. Always lie with your legs stretched out, one knee bent and your weight supported by your elbows. This allows you to make eye contact, sip drinks and stare mysteriously out to sea, whilst remaining as long and lean as….a supermodel.

If you've got a dodgy **bottom**, swap your bikini pants for a pair of swimshorts or generously cut hot pants. Never buy bikini bottoms with tie-sides – they'll cut into your side flab like cheese wire. Avoid high fashion bikinis like the Burberry's check number – you'll look self-conscious and dated.

Never wear thongs, however fabulous your bottom. Less is more doesn't apply here … low-rent and vulgar does. Conversely, don't assume that a one-piece swimming costume will cover all sins and flatter all bodies. They tend to emphasise every bulge because they pull so tightly over the trunk.

Invest in a splendidly forgiving tankini. These Calvin Klein pioneered vest and hipster pant combos are très wearable – sharp, structured, sporty and chic. They're designed to sit, flatter and stay put. Definitely the kindest cut.

If big **arms** are your problem, opt for a split-sleeve T-shirt that thins the sides of the arm, an off-the-shoulder top with sleeves or an eighties-style slash-neck sweatshirt that slops sexily over your bronzed shoulders. Do not wrap a jumper of any description around your shoulders before sauntering out – it will only draw attention to the area you're trying to disguise.

Elongate your **legs** by wrapping up in a sarong and choosing wedges over flip-flops for that three-inch head start. Always put your wedges on before you stand up and make them the last things you take off when you lie down.

If your problem is your **stomach**, or your entire body feels bloated and doesn't want to go 'on show' then close your eyes and say a little thank you that the kaftan has re-emerged as the hot style and sun essential after lying dormant for thirty years.

11

How to look great whatever your lifestyle

Models with great potential often drop out of international modelling because they find the hectic lifestyle impossible to maintain. The profession demands that they regularly commute between the four major fashion cities of New York, Paris, Milan and London where the world's leading fashion designers, magazines and photographers are based.

The relentless, non-stop travel with constant time changes, means irregular sleeping and eating patterns which can lead to stress and exhaustion – affecting a girl's well-being and appearance.

This gruelling pace intensifies several times a year when the fashion designers show their collections in the four major key cities. The top girls are booked by the designers to show their creations on the cat-walk, and are fought over by the glossy magazines to be photographed wearing the clothes on their pages.

Dashing from one designer show to another, last-minute rehearsals, quick changes and inevitable after-show parties needs extraordinary stamina and resilience. Often the photographic shoots take place late at night as every magazine wants to be the first to publish the star garments of the collections.

'You're never allowed to be tired', sighs Kate Moss and unless a top model paces herself sensibly and follows strict regular regimes for survival, it is possible for her to easily become mentally and physically exhausted.

How to fly long distance and arrive jet fresh

- On board change into comfy baggy trousers and a long-sleeved cotton top.

- Swap high heels for cashmere socks.

- Take off make-up and apply Guerlain's Midnight Secret travel stick – a serum that mainlines into tired skin.

- Fill a two-litre bottle of mineral water with a sachet of multi-vitamin powder.

- Surround yourself with books, magazines and a pashmina (has-been fashion item, best ever travel blanket).

- Set your watch for the time of your destination.

- When airborne, drink heaps of water and don't even think about alcohol.

- Moisturise your face and hands.

- Eat only the vegetarian menu you have ordered in advance.

- Walk up and down the aisle and stretch as much as possible.

- When standing (waiting for the loo) stretch your legs by slowly bending back one knee at a time. Reach back and catch hold of your foot, pulling it towards your body. Hold for a slow count of five, and then repeat with the other foot.

- Spritz water on your face; models swear by Evian or Vichy sprays. Helena Christensen's favourite is Remo Facial Mist, which she picks up from Sydney's most fashionable store of the same name.

- Discourage fellow travellers from chatting by saying you're exhausted and must get some rest. Say goodnight sweetly, insert earplugs and put on an eyemask.

- Before landing, do some stretches, clean teeth, comb hair and change back into fresh travel clothes. Apply more moisturiser and a pair of sunglasses.

- Never think what time it is where you came from.

- Don't go to bed if you arrive during the day, however tired you are. You'll wake up in the middle of the night.

- Unpack. Have a shower. Go for a walk in the park. Have a swim. Keep busy. Early night – fall into bed.

Sitting for hours on a plane with no possibility of exercise, and mediocre food presented at irregular intervals, plays havoc with your digestive system. Irritable bowel syndrome is rife among the models who travel the world non-stop.

When I was modelling I worked with many girls who overcame this problem by sprinkling linseeds on their food. The high absorption capacity of linseeds provides the body with bulk which helps to maintain digestive regularity, and the mucins provide a protective layer for the intestines. Two dessertspoons of organic linseeds on your cereal, yoghurt, soup or salad each day keeps your system healthy the natural, gentle way.

During times of high pressure most models take a daily multi-vitamin as an insurance policy. Extra vitamin C is also wise and the models' favourite brand is Berocca, a lozenge added to water which makes a delicious tropical tasting drink. It contains 1000 mg of vitamin C plus B complex – making it the perfect skin repairer, immunity booster and all round reviver for hectic lifestyles. Available worldwide.

Letting off steam

It's hardly surprising that when the fashion collections are over, models reward their hard work with some fun, which includes a few… er drops of champagne and one or two cigarettes. I remember on the last day of the Paris collections a gaggle of us would always descend on a night club and dance with each other till dawn (ignoring strange looks from jet-set gigolos). Then we would move on to the early morning food market, where the porters would give us delicious hot onion soup until the sun came up.

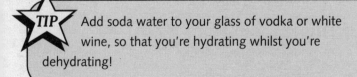

> **TIP** If your feet are killing you in those ridiculously high Jimmy Choos and you badly need to dance, rub neat vodka all over your feet. The vodka numbs the pain and you'll be dancing till dawn.

Post-party remedies

When restraint goes out of the window we have to pay the price. Of course we know by now the only two key ingredients that cure a hangover are water and time – but we always forget the former and never have enough time for the latter.

> **TIP** Add soda water to your glass of vodka or white wine, so that you're hydrating whilst you're dehydrating!

Avoid a truly nasty hangover by taking Silicol Gel before you drink alcohol. One tablespoon lines the entire stomach and intestine with a protective layer of natural silicic acid which neutralises and removes toxins from the gut. Take another spoonful before bed to ensure minimal damage.

If you forget your Silicol Gel, the best hangover remedy ever is Nux Vomica homeopathic tablets taken the second you experience hangover symptoms. Take 4 tablets of the 6 potency three times daily, or two tablets of the 30 potency three times daily. Take with buckets of water. Both available at health food stores and chemists worldwide. Brand names may differ.

> **TIP** The last six things to remember on party night:
> 1. Remove all your make-up.
> 2. Apply a night cream or serum.
> 3. Apply a night-time eye cream.
> 4. Drink a pint of water.
> 5. Take a vitamin C tablet.
> 6. Apply some fake tan (could be dangerous if very unsteady).

Ponder the question: Is a hangover the wrath of grapes? Ha!

Part Three
Style

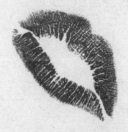

Whilst working as a model for Vogue with photographer Helmut Newton, I once asked him how he came to choose his models. 'I look for a certain defiance, and good posture is important. Nonchalance, and that indefinable way in which a girl wears the clothes rather than allowing the clothes to wear her', he said. 'It's that elusive thing called style.' Blimey, I thought. What on earth am I doing here, being only expert at 'le style slob' at the time. It must have been my defiance.

'It's a dangerous thing to be too modern; one is apt to grow old-fashioned quite suddenly.'
Oscar Wilde

12

The difference between fashion and style

So what exactly is style? We know it when we see it but how do we define style and more importantly, how do we acquire it? Well, like Oscar Wilde, I think being stylish owes very little to the latest fashion. You can be very fashionable without having any style and you can be stylish without ever being fashionable. Money does not buy you instant style.

Kate Moss' close friend, actress Sadie Frost says,

> *'I think it's a lot sexier when someone looks a bit unkempt. You think to yourself "What were they up to last night?" People are more attractive when they look comfortable with their bodies.'*

Creating the desired effect of nonchalance takes a some-what determined effort, but it is an art form that can be learned. The first major investment you make should be a full-length mirror, positioned near lots of natural light and preferably where you can see yourself from all angles, including the back.

This may seem brutal, but an honest, overall image of yourself is essential to eliminate the 'in-denial' size 10 obsession; the too-short trouser leg and the 'God you can see my knickers through this fabric' moment whilst catching your reflection in a shop window.

Trying too hard (TTH)

TTH is an abbreviation often used by stylists on fashion shoots where over-gilding the lily (unless ironic) is the enemy of cool and generally a far worse crime than not trying too hard (NTTH).

Away from the camera, it's virtually impossible to ever see a supermodel looking as though she's TTH. The very nature of her work means she dresses down as a reaction to wearing countless garments for a living. Slipping on her tenth Gucci outfit of the day means nothing beyond the fact that it's the last on the rack to be photographed before she can go home.

> *'When I see someone completely dressed in labels, it makes me think there's something missing in their self-esteem and somehow they have to compensate. Although I love working with Jean Paul Gaultier and feel great in his*

designs, my own clothes are now far less crazy and frivolous than when I was a medical student.

I suppose, as a model, I care less about the image of the clothes than before. I don't care if what I wear is the latest design or that by next season it's past it.' **Catherine Hurley**

Those chic young women gliding down the road dressed head-to-toe in designer labels are never models, but the trophy wives of rich men, fashionistas, and women who make their living from fashion, such as stylists and fashion editors. Supermodels wear jeans, T-shirts and a comfortable, anonymous jacket and don't look 'on show' when they are going about their business. They leave the dressing up for when they want to be photographed at 'occasion' bashes.

How to avoid trying too hard:

- *Never buy the latest ugly designer handbag simply to be the first. You may as well have fashion victim tattooed on your forehead.*
- *Go easy on the jewellery. It's amazing how cheap too much expensive gold can look.*
- *Never buy leather trousers in any colour. They make your thighs, stomach and bottom look twice their size.*

- *Don't even think about culottes, pinafore dresses, knickerbockers, batwing sleeves, circular skirts, pleats or anything 'babydoll' unless you're under 18 or attempting a so-wrong-it's-right look.*
- *Never sport a label top-to-toe. Mix high-street, designer and maybe vintage.*
- *Don't wear an outfit where everything is completely new. Clothes need to have soul.*
- *Never look too groomed. Loosen up, dance around, shake your hair, undo a button.*

How to discover your true style

Despite having access to any label in the world, Kate Moss always puts her own spin on the way she looks. She knows exactly what suits her, is never a slave to fashion trends and has the utter confidence to be herself. Kate has a knack of knowing how to dress for every occasion and the ability to throw on a mix of designer, high-street and vintage clothes that always works.

When she does evening 'glamour' she always gets the proportions right, often wearing a simple, slinky one-tone dress, teamed with strappy stilettos and a beautiful vintage handbag. She always wears sexy shoes (you hardly ever see her in trainers) and this elegant yet eclectic style is reflected in her favourite designers – Alexander McQueen, Vivienne Westwood, Helmut Lang and Versace.

This individuality and confidence with clothes is something all top models acquire from wearing thousands of garments a year and having to make them come alive. Photographers, fashion editors and designers are brutally honest about which garments suit each girl (and which don't) and models learn over time what's best for them and, from stylists, how to wear them.

It's important to build up a wardrobe that expresses your personality. It's no good dressing in tailored classics if you're really a romantic and long for velvet and frills, or doing the hippy peasant look if you love androgynous clothes.

Choosing bright colours and patterns if you're an introvert, or dressing in three tones of grey if you long to be the life and soul of the party, is never going to work. Approach your wardrobe from the premise that it has to suit you, not you it. Your style is your trademark; it reflects your character and lifestyle. It's your very own sartorial signature.

TIP The knack of walking well in very high heels is to walk on the balls of your feet, not your heels.

Elle Macpherson's lifestyle is jet-set international – she has four magnificent homes around the world and her personal style reflects this – polished, elegant, and groomed and Valentino is, unsurprisingly, her favourite designer.

Yasmin Le Bon is married to a musician and her look is

more 'romantic rock and roll', favouring denim and the occasional pretty forties tea dress. Jeans, Ossie Clark and Voyage are her favourites and she was one of the first girls to be seen in kid's T-shirts and cut-off denim skirts. She's also one of the few girls who can wear Day-Glo colours and still look amazing.

> *'I've been wearing vintage clothes since I was a teenager. My mother has a vintage clothes shop in Denmark and I love the beautiful fabrics. If I buy a designer garment it's never because of the label, but because I love it. I guess my style is a bit bohemian — I enjoy shopping at markets. I save high heels for dressing up and just like to feel comfortable during the day. I simply wear what feels good at the time.'*
>
> *Helena Christensen*

Claudia Schiffer is another model who loves mixing old with new and she enjoys nothing more than rummaging around bargain bins in shops. She says one of her best ever buys was a vintage leather jacket she spotted in Portobello Road, London, which she swears she'll keep forever. Chloe jeans are another favourite of Claudia's and it's a relief to know that she finds really good jeans hard to find – like the rest of us.

It isn't uncommon to continue to dress according to the decade of your heyday, whilst believing you're still of-the-moment. A good way to avoid image time warp is to assess your style of dressing every ten years. Keeping the same hairstyle long-term can also make you look older, because the face changes but the hair stays the same emphasising the ageing face rather than disguising it.

You can't wear that at your age

- *Twenties. Wean yourself away from cheap, stretchy fabrics, piercings, crop tops. Think Miu Miu. Never attempt Armani suits, Hermès scarves or beige.*
- *Thirties. Say goodbye to mini skirts, plastic jewellery, spangly stuff, and hair bobbles. Think Zara and Gucci. No long jackets, floral skirts or Jean Muir.*
- *Forties. Au revoir gingham, customised denim, Luella, long hair and vintage. Think DKNY, cashmere and Jimmy Choo. Say no to leisure pants.*
- *Fifties. Relax, you know what suits you. Put on your good jewellery and marvel at the wonderful character in your face. That's your signature style.*

The low-down on handbags

Just how many handbags does a girl need these days? The key pieces in your wardrobe should be an expensive looking investment bag that makes you feel well-groomed, a stylish bag for summer, a sexy evening bag, a fun bag that makes you smile, and a great in-flight/travel bag that opens easily at the top.

A black leather bag is too heavy for summer. Soft, creamy fabrics like pale suede, printed and embroidered cottons, and straw or raffia work best. Forget the 'matching bag and shoes' idea and think of bags and shoes as separate accessories – jazz up an outfit with funky shoes or an unusually shaped bag (not both) and balance a wild outfit with a simple clutch bag.

Go for the Russian doll effect when you go to work. Carry a large tote bag, but keep a smart but smaller handbag inside it, that you can take out during the day. That way you can leave all your other stuff (gym kit, magazines etc) in your large bag, under your desk.

To be suitably dressed – taking into account the occasion and the people you're sharing it with – is an important part of feeling comfortable and confident with your style. One of my many fatal fashion faux-pas over the years illustrates 'how-not-to-do-it'.

I was working with two other models on location in St Moritz in Switzerland and the Shah of Iran was staying in the same hotel and asked us to join him for dinner. The other two models wore Christian Dior and Yves St Laurent dresses but I decided to remain under-whelmed by this regal invitation, reflecting my political views at the time, and wore early Liam Gallagher – a pair of jeans and a kind of old anorak.

The Shah was charming to me, but I knew I'd got it wrong. I should have refused the invitation or respected the situation by dressing appropriately. Later he sent me an enormous tin of Iranian caviar, probably because he thought I needed feeding up for my next protest rally.

The moral of the story is to never dress outrageously unless you have the total confidence to carry it off. Be different but not enough to feel uncomfortable or to be insulting to your host.

13

What clothes to buy from where

It takes great skill to mix designer, high-street and vintage clothes but is well worth the effort if you get it right and understand how to balance the diversity of influences.

Designer

Expensive to purchase, making impulse buying an even worse idea than usual. Never shop for designer clothes when you're in an odd mood – when you're a bit depressed and need a lift – and feel you have to buy something. Or when you have those strange highs where you kid yourself that the garment you are about to buy will look fabulous and be very useful when you lose a stone, get that perfect holiday tan, or go to all those parties you know you'll be invited to.

Never be frightened to enter designer establishments – they need you – and don't ever be intimidated by the assistants. The good ones are really helpful and explain the designer's philosophy to you by showing you how to build up 'the look'. The bad, snotty ones are idiots because they've possibly just kissed goodbye to a hefty commission by alienating you. Remember to always check your rear view when trying on clothes, and if the changing room has distorting mirrors, the closer you are, the more realistic the image.

The idea when shopping for designer clothes is to buy one key item that is so beautiful, it's worth every penny you pay. Designer scores over high-street in the quality of the fabric and in the cut of the garment. So it makes more sense to buy one sensational jacket, dress, suit or coat than basics like tops, shirts and jeans, which are copied well by the high-street shops.

Unless you're loaded, never buy anything faddy from a designer store. Pay proportionately for how often the item will be worn. You'll feel better spending a small fortune on a coat for everyday than an evening top you'll wear three times a year.

It's a good idea to venture into designer stores at the beginning of every season to look, absorb and get a taste for the new designs and colours. That way you'll get a feel for what you should be wearing and you can either look for cheaper high-street versions or adapt and customise what you already have, or buy the one key versatile item that will bring your entire wardrobe up to date.

High-street
··

A few years ago fashion editors wouldn't have been seen dead in a high-street version of a garment, but today they compete to find the best seasonal must-have. The quality and style of high-street clothes is better than ever and even die-hard style queens aren't stupid enough to pay heaps of money for an identical designer version.

The young high-street chains are now producing fabulous versions of those designer looks we all covet but can't afford. Top designers like Gucci and Prada are favourite points of inspiration, but if you want the best pieces you'll have to be quick because they sell the stock within hours of it going on the shelves, making it scarily similar to designer wear in the popularity stakes.

There are certain rules for successful high-street shopping. Steer clear of highly patterned, outrageously designed garments. Trends that weren't flattering on the catwalk are never going to work in real life, especially in cheaper fabrics.

The trick is to be selective. Opt for designer-inspired pieces that aren't too tricksy, badly made or garish. A Versace-style dress from a cheap chain is not a good idea. Versace can be tacky enough, so a copy with a dodgier cut will definitely not cut it.

The top five classic fashion buys:

1. Cashmere Jumpers. Feel and look delicious and won't scream last season. Realistic prices if you look carefully.
2. The Little Black Dress. Black is always back; the best investment a girl can make.
3. Well-cut Trousers. It's the bottom line.
4. Winter Overcoat. It will never date if you choose classic and simple.
5. Jeans. If they fit well, buy buy buy.

Vintage

Most models now possess at least one item of clothing that is older than they are. Old is fresh. This came about as a reaction to 'designeritis' where the same designer clothes are seen all over the world at the beginning of the season and no-one can be individual. And because vintage clothes are so beautifully made and have a soul. They're the nearest thing young people have to haute couture.

According to Virginia Bates, who owns one of the best vintage clothes shops in London, it was Helena Christensen who started the ball rolling back in the early nineties when she started buying and wearing antique slip dresses and cardigans.

'Helena was doing the shows in London and Naomi saw what she was wearing, and suddenly all the girls backstage were wearing my frocks.'
Virginia Bates

Wearing vintage can be tricky and should never be worn by anyone old enough to have worn it the first time around. Never wear it from head-to-toe – keep your shoes and jewellery modern – or people will think you've stepped out of a period drama. Think in terms of buying a one-off piece rather than a particular label. Mix hard with feminine – a denim jacket with a forties tea dress, a vintage Oriental jacket with jeans, a high-street cardigan with a vintage Chanel dress or Kate Moss' current favourite look of faded denim jeans with an elaborate vintage top.

Before you buy vintage, check for underarm staining and give the garment a quick sniff, as even dry-cleaning often won't remove decades of body odour. Watch out for moths and don't dance with anyone too boisterous.

Yves St Laurent couture from the sixties and seventies is now worth a serious fortune. The ready-to-wear Rive Gauche range is worth less, but is still collectable. Very early Christian Dior, Elsa Schiaparelli, sixties Balenciaga and anything from twenties and thirties Coco Chanel regularly fetch thousands. Word has it that John Galliano and Vivienne Westwood will be hot next and in the future Alexander McQueen will be super collectable.

Every major city has its vintage designer stores and part of the fun is to discover one that nobody else has found, making the variety of choice and price to your advantage.

Established auction houses like Sotheby's now have vintage sales several times a year. For the very best websites for buying designer clothes from a few seasons' ago at discount prices, see Resources.

How to shop in the sales

- Don't buy anything that isn't you. We buy impulsively to make us feel like different people. But if the disparity between what you buy and your real self is too wide, you'll feel worse not better.

- Ask yourself whether you would have wanted this garment before the price was reduced.

- Never buy clothes you intend to diet into. You'll want to buy new clothes to celebrate your new shape.

- That 'great buy' is in the sale for a good reason. No-one wanted it.

- Never shop when you're hungry – you'll either buy too much to compensate or nothing because you're too distracted. Pack a snack box to keep you going.

- Before you buy a wacky purchase, imagine someone else wearing what you're about to buy and ask yourself what you would think of them.

- Think about the fabric. If you travel a lot you don't need clothes that crease in a suitcase. If you have kids, you need machine washable clothes.

■ Don't buy anything because it's so 'original'. The reason it hasn't been designed yet is it simply doesn't work.

■ If you find something you like, walk away and give yourself ten minutes to think about it. Ask yourself, 'Do I really need this?' Then pay for it in cash. It's much more painful passing over the notes than having your credit card swiped.

Mastering the sales and snapping up pieces you will wear over and over again is always satisfying. The trick is to know what looks good on you and to stick to it, instead of shopping recreationally and randomly. Buy pieces that will take you through to next season and possibly through to next winter. Classics, of course, are timeless.

Five accessories to buy in the sales that won't date

1. *Designer Shoes.* Buy classic Ginas and Manolos and you'll be wearing them 5 years from now.
2. *Leather Belt.* Improves with age.
3. *Tote Bag.* Simple classic shape in leather.
4. *Leather Boots.* Flat, knee-highs; never around in shops when you're looking for them.
5. *Lingerie.* Stock up; you won't feel guilty if it's reduced.

14

Flattering fashion tricks

A full-length mirror, where you can also check side and back views, is essential. It's impossible to assess your silhouette without one. Ask a friend what she honestly thinks of your posture and, if she's not brimming with compliments, aim to improve it with the help of yoga, Pilates or simple stretching exercises. Good posture is the best trick ever for gaining extra height.

The walk that models perform on the catwalk is not simply for show. It actually lengthens their legs. This is what you do:

1. Keep your shoulders back.

2. Hold your head high.

3. Push your hips forward when walking.

4. Place one foot directly in front of the other.

5. Push your pelvis very slightly forward – and lead with the hips.

To look tall and slim

··

- Wear one solid colour from head-to-toe.

- Keep your outline sleek and unfussy.

- Choose a pair of tailored trousers that are cut a little too long for you and add very high heels.

- Wear flat-fronted, boot-cut trousers with a side zip. Avoid pleated fronts and flaps on pockets.

- A-line skirts are slimming and work even better if they are cut on the bias. Inverted pleats (one or many) also slim your shape.

- A tailored jacket should have skinny sleeves set high in the arm-hole. Avoid raglan sleeves.

- Choose a jacket that doesn't button exactly on the waist – a little above or below is best.

- A jacket/trousers with vertical stripes will add those extra inches.

- Always wear socks or pop socks in the same colour as your trousers.

- Dresses cut on the bias of the cloth (wool, silk, jersey) slim you if you buy a size that skims rather than clings.

TIP Do the Camel Toe Test before you buy tight trousers. Sit down in them, bend down and walk around. If the trousers don't fit, they'll find your centre parting and reveal your crotch.

Legs

- Never wear tights under trousers. They act as a magnet making the fabric cling. Thighs look twice their size.

- Make sure bare legs are fake tanned. An even skin tone makes them appear slimmer and shapelier.

- Dust blusher or bronzing powder in a narrow line up your shin and thigh to accentuate the bone for a slimming effect.

- High-heeled, strappy sandals worn with bare legs, elongate the legs.

- Black opaque tights are the most flattering.

- A skirt with a small side slit is the best shape for a fuller leg.

- If you've got fat legs, wear high boots with skirts and dresses. Never wear shoes with ankle straps; they cut the leg in two.

- To make ankles appear thinner, wear slightly heavier shoes.

Big bust

∙∙∙

- A sleeveless, thin, ribbed turtle neck top will minimise your curves.

- Big bosoms look best in deep v- or sweetheart necklines or a wrap-around top

- Never wear anything with a high, round neck.

- Twin-sets look frumpy on big breasts. Try a v-neck cardigan over a reverse collar shirt instead.

- Wear dark colours on the top half and light shades below. Dark colours recede while light ones stand out.

- Avoid double-breasted jackets. Go for slim and tailored single-breasted jackets that don't button too high.

- Choose tailored shirts and blouses rather than full ones.

TIP Before you go out, sit down in what you're wearing and look in a mirror. You may be surprised by what it reveals. If it all rolls and pulls around your middle, think again.

Short-waisted

· ·

- The best jacket shape for you is hip length or longer.

- Double-breasted is okay but single-breasted is better because it elongates the torso.

- A high, round neck will make your upper body look longer.

- Avoid patch pockets and pockets with a strong horizontal seam.

- Look for slash pockets that are sewn into the jacket at a slight angle below the waist.

- Choose a skirt that hits the knees.

- Trousers should be low-slung, flat-fronted and straight-legged.

- Wear T-shirts and tops that are slim-fitting and never tuck them in.

- Reverse all the above procedures if you're long-waisted.

'I'm extremely tall so the most important thing is to have the waist in the right place. I stick to basics — plain clothes, no patterns, in a range of colours. Quite simple really. I love cotton because natural materials feel so good. My favourite casual look is jeans and a white T-shirt.' **Catherine Hurley**

Why choosing the right colours is so important

Choosing a garment in the wrong colour will destroy the hard work you put into your make-up, hair and clothes. Wearing a flattering shade will enhance all your attributes.

It is a rare woman who can successfully wear a bright colour head-to-toe if she is over the age of 25 and away from the beach. On the whole it's best to keep bright colour to details like lip colour, T-shirts, jackets, scarves, shoes, bags and belts.

Over co-ordinating your colours will make you look like a circus escapee. Keep the Christian Lacroix dream outfit for your dreams, even if you have a strong love of colour, pattern and a sheer, no-fear approach to clash.

> *'I love Schiaparelli pink and used to wear it often — but your skin tone changes as you get older and stronger colours wipe you out.'*
>
> *Fiona Campbell-Walter*

This look is high-maintenance and simply doesn't work off the cat-walk unless it's done with brilliant panache and the wearer has a radiant complexion, hair like a dream, and stays looking as fresh as a daisy all day/night.

On the other hand playing it too safe can be just as bad. For example, beige and camel shades can make pale brunettes look sick, and white on an ivory-complexioned blonde also makes you head for the medicine chest.

Wearing the wrong shade of grey can make your skin look even greyer and even black, that old perennial basic, can be too hard for some skin tones, who should try navy instead.

If you often feel you look drained in whatever you wear, try holding different coloured garments up to your face when you next go shopping and be open-minded about what they reveal. Ask a reliable girlfriend to give you an honest appraisal of the colours you wear and whether she thinks they flatter you.

Even if black suits you, make sure you keep it matt. Avoid daytime outfits in black that shine (often made from blends of polyester and viscose). A white trim (of T-shirt, collar or cuff) between you and your black sweater is more flattering during the day than wearing black next to your skin. And black for summer? Tread carefully. It looks best with a tan or gothic with a pale skin.

- Colours that Expand: White, yellow, orange, purple, lime green and pink

- Colours that Camouflage: Neutrals and pastels

- Colours that Minimise: Black, navy and grey

TIP Remember that patterns with a dark background are more slimming than those with a pale or neutral base.

15

How to look incredibly rich on very little money

The alternative to the combination 'designer/vintage/high-street' look that Kate and Claudia love to bits is the rich, international style of dressing that Elle Macpherson and Cindy Crawford do so well.

Their effortless chic and pared down style make other women green with envy. Nothing appears to jar or jangle; everything works and goes together to form the perfect capsule wardrobe. No fuss – high luxe.

This look is easier to emulate than you might imagine but you have to know the rules. There are three areas that give the game away: jewellery, bag and shoes.

Arm candy

To be a rich player you must keep jewellery to a serious minimum, except for the presence of an expensive watch.

This is your only major expense in the entire 'looking rich' fandango but will carry you through, and people won't notice the cheap bits.

Buy the most expensive watch you can afford. It should be instantly recognisable as a quality watch – say a Cartier tank or a Rolex. It's no good buying a limited design Frank Muller – only serious fashionistas will recognise it, defeating the object.

Save up for your watch by sacrificing nail-bar manicures (more about those later), eating out less, not buying so many skin-care items, and never buying 'fun' jewellery - safe in the knowledge that your eternal timepiece will give you the ultimate, luxurious satisfaction every time you gaze at your wrist.

Pawn shops are good places to pick up expensive watches at bargain prices. Auction houses have regular vintage designer watch sales and Duty Free shops in places like Kuala Lumpur often sell the real thing at rock bottom prices. Failing that, there are some excellent copies around (especially in Hong Kong) and you can always move your arm around a lot, making it difficult to focus on the fake.

Bags of money

Your bag should whisper 'good taste'. A leather Kelly or Birkin bag by Hermès is the kind of thing, though not the kind of price at several thousand smackers for a new one. There are some excellent copies around, and you could get lucky in an obscure vintage shop. Forget Louis Vuitton or Burberry, real or fake – too many cheap, nasty copies have demeaned the real thing.

A summer bag is easier to cheat. As long as it's light and pretty, you'll get by but don't wear a heavy leather bag with summer clothes and don't wear a structured bag with unstructured clothing.

Are they Choos?

Look for good high-street copies of designer shoes. The less shoe there is, the easier it is to fake. High-heeled, high-street strappy sandals don't look that different to those by Sergio Rossi, once you're wearing them.

Never wear black shoes with light clothes or tapered leg trousers with court shoes or boots – wear chunky soled shoes. Only wear high heels with mid-calf pencil skirts and wear only flat shoes, kitten mules or boots with bias-cut long skirts.

The right stuff

Resist the impulse to be sartorially witty or off-beat – it doesn't work in this refined world. Colours are always muted and 'tasteful'. Think Park Avenue Princess in different hues of one shade – caramel cashmere combined with honey, cream, oatmeal and a splash of Colmans. Or Jerry Hall, lunching with friends wearing a black polo-neck jumper, black slacks and loafers with Butler & Wilson grey pearls.

Shiny fabrics never work, day or night – and a cheap, tailored jacket is something of an oxymoron. Don't even waste your time looking – they have nasty fabric, cheap stitching and are never well-hung. Instead, look for last year's Marc Jacobs or Helmut Lang tailored jacket at your poshest charity shop or on the Web. (See Resources.) Wear it with Tod's (type) loafers, jeans and a high-street T-shirt and cashmere sweater.

You could look like this for years – with an inexpensive little black evening dress and some white linen (neither show up cheap stitching) thrown in. The main advantage of the rich look is that you need very few clothes and accessories – it's timeless quality not quantity that counts.

- Invest in the finest fabric you can afford.

- Opt for simple shapes and neutral colours.

- Resolve to buy less but buy better.

A word about cashmere. There is nothing, absolutely nothing, to beat it compared to other types of wool. It feels so wonderful next to your skin that, once you're hooked, it's impossible to wear anything else. And it never looks tired. And it always looks rich.

Of course, a cashmere sweater costs more than one made from Shetland wool, but the gap is narrowing. I found the most sensational cashmere sweater at a large branch of one of the major supermarkets recently – great colour range, brilliant simple design – for virtually the same price as an average woollen jumper.

Looking rich checklist

- *Posh handbag – cheap brolly.*
- *Chic shoes – budget tights.*
- *Designer watch – no 'fun' jewellery.*
- *Expensive jacket – cheap T-shirt.*
- *Top haircut – home manicure.*
- *Designer sunglasses – cheap flip-flops.*
- *Signature scent – supermarket body lotion.*

How to smell rich

Your smell says a lot about you. Your style can be shattered by a sharp, stinky scent. The ubiquitous, mass-produced perfumes you buy at Duty Free have no place on the pulse points of the seriously well-heeled. They prefer a signature scent, mixed specifically to their requirements by a French perfumery at great expense.

This innovative approach to fragrance is catching on. More and more of us want unusual, unique subtle smells we can call our own. Customising our own concoctions by mixing different scents together would be sacrilege to an expert parfumier, but it can be done with great success. A friend of mine mixes Jo Malone's Lime Basil and Mandarin cologne with pure musk oil and it smells wonderful on her.

The only scent I wear is a mixture of three fragrances from L'Artisan Parfumeur, which my romantic and enterprising partner customised for me as a totally original birthday present several years ago. The formula is $\frac{7}{16}$ Fig; $\frac{7}{16}$ Vetiver and $\frac{2}{16}$ Mimosa and the result is so staggeringly fab that, every time I wear it, at least three people ask me what it is. There goes my best-kept beauty secret. The things I do for my publisher!

L'Artisan Parfumeur is a French perfume boutique in Chelsea, London (there are 25 of them across France) that stock their own unusual scents. See Resources for more details.

> *'I don't really wear perfumes but I love using essential oils like Rose, Lavender or Sandalwood — they are calming and smell lovely.'*
> **Christy Turlington**

The effect of smelling good can be quickly ruined by over-kill. If you tend to be heavy-handed with the spray, opt for eau de toilette, which isn't as strong as perfume or eau de parfum. Your scent should not be smelt beyond arm's length and the best way to avoid over-kill is to spray the air in front of you, then walk through the cloud.

Three supermodels who love Guerlain

Shalimar *'I'm very classic when it comes to perfume.'*
Carla Bruni
Vetiver *'I like the way male fragrances smell on me.'*
Elle Macpherson
Vol de Nuit *'My true favourites are old French perfumes.'* **Ines de la Fressange**

Getting nailed

Long red talons, elaborate painted falsies and 'sculptured extensions' may be suitably high maintenance, but they seriously don't cut it in luxury land where they are considered somewhat taste-deficient.

Nails simply need to look unnoticeable – clean, a decent shape, pushed down cuticles and a coat of neutralish varnish. It's no big deal and, for the life of me, I don't understand why this can't be done at home.

When I first heard about nail bars I thought, 'What an enterprising idea – somewhere to meet a girlfriend after work and have a drink and a manicure at the same time – a sort of pleasurable multi-tasking scenario.' But sadly they're just boring places where a manicurist pushes back your cuticles, whizzes a brush over your nails, makes mindless conversation about holidays and charges you a disproportionate amount of cash.

Frankly, the time saved could be put to better use, and the money could go towards your watch or a good haircut or be invested in a long-term money saver – like permanent laser hair removal. Now there's something worth spending money on!

> **TIP** For hands that look smooth enough to have been lounging on a yacht for years, keep two types of hand cream next to every set of taps. Each time you wash your hands follow with a day cream containing an SPF or a richer cream for evening use.

16

How to edit your wardrobe on a regular basis

At the start of every season, try on the clothes you have for that season in front of your full-length mirror and ask yourself the following questions:

- Does this outfit make me look long and lean and flatter my body shape?

- Is this garment fashionable enough to wear for another season?

- Do I feel positive and confident when I wear this?

- Does the colour enhance my complexion and hair?

If the answer is yes, place in the 'keep' pile. If you're not sure put in the 'maybe' pile.

If your reply is:

- I didn't wear this once last year but it might come in useful for …

- It's falling to pieces but it reminds me of …

- It's a bit small, but it's designer and it cost the earth …

place in the 'give to best friend/cousin/charity shop' pile. Be ruthless. There is simply no point in cluttering up your wardrobe with items you will never wear. Chuck out the 'maybe' pile.

Take the 'keep' pile and accessorise each outfit with what's available from your shoe, jewellery, scarf, and shirt department. If your accessories flatter the garment and look fresh and up-to-date, sketch or photograph the outfit and its appropriate accessories and tape it inside your wardrobe for permanent quick reference.

The number of sketches/photos you end up with will reveal your shockingly low selection of main garments and pitifully out-of-touch collection of accessories – or disclose that you have more than enough stylish outfits for the forthcoming season and simply need a new pair of shoes and a few T-shirts.

Make a list of what's lacking in your wardrobe – maybe you never seem to have enough everyday tops – or you have an item that suits you, but you have nothing to wear with it. Put what you need on the list and shop specifically for those items. Culling and updating your wardrobe in this way means your clothes always have your trademark – a continuity of style that's uniquely yours. Panic and impulse buying will become experiences from your distant past.

Viewing and looking after your clothes

For years I never really cared about how I kept my clothes. Most things were flung to the back of the wardrobe and dry-cleaned when I remembered. It seemed perfectly natural for me to rummage around in a blind panic for a pair of shoes to go with an outfit. But that was before my humiliating horror story, some years ago.

I was meeting friends for dinner and as I made my entrance down the stairs to the mega-cool, celebrity-packed dining room, I noticed the entire restaurant was looking at me – or rather at my feet. I looked down to see a pair of black tights trailing from my left trouser leg.

I'd stripped off the trousers and tights together after their last outing and they'd become lovingly inter-twined – and I'd slithered back into the trousers oblivious to the lurking hosiery.

Well that was enough humiliation to make me change my sluttish behaviour overnight and I've never looked back. Giving your wardrobe a good work-out literally changes your life. It's the ultimate satisfying experience – much better than shopping.

You are going to re-design and re-organise your wardrobe so that you see everything at once!

- Put all your clothes in your wardrobe and keep drawers for underwear, nightwear and exercise gear.

- Make more room in your wardrobe by adding rails and putting away summer clothes in winter, including shoes. Pack away and place under your bed in suitcases.

- Invest in some new hangers specifically designed for trousers, skirts, dresses, jackets and coats.

- Hang as much as possible including T-shirts, tops and light jumpers for visual access and to minimise creasing.

- Place the hangers the same way round, so that the entire wardrobe looks like a smart shop.

- Never place more than one item on a hanger.

- Throw out T-shirts that have become dull from washing.

- Hang coloured clothes together as complete outfits.

- Group all your clothes by shade, placing pinks next to reds next to magentas etc.

- Hang neutrals – black, beige and white basics in their separate categories of trousers, tops, jackets, coats and skirts mixing textures and fabrics together to keep it interesting.

- Put belts on tie racks or over the hooks of hangers.

- Hang accessories on nails inside your wardrobe doors. Hang necklaces and bracelets next to evening bags in the same colours.

- Wash your jumpers regularly – moths love stale bits of food.

TIP Stop angora sweaters moulting with a quick spritz
of hairspray

- The very best thing to keep moths away is conkers.

- Dry-clean big jumpers at the end of winter and keep in
plastic bags.

- Have your cashmere items laundered and packed in tissue
paper when storing long-term.

- Make sure your shoes are clean and the heels don't need
repairing before putting them back in the wardrobe.

- Buy lots of shoe trees and always use them as soon as you
take off your shoes, while the leather or fabric is still warm.

- Keep special shoes in boxes with a photo of each pair
attached to the box for quick visual access.

- Always put your clothes away at night after checking
whether they need cleaning (and check for rogue tights).

- Tidy your wardrobe once a week, placing things in their
right order.

Supermodel repair secrets

In every major city there's a well-kept sartorial secret
that's worth its weight in gold. Quite often models will
divulge their insider knowledge with the same conspirato-

rial air as when discovering a great masseur, facialist or hairstylist.

I'm talking about an alterations genius. Someone who can make that size 16 trouser suit you couldn't resist in the sale fit a size 10 body with ease and flair. The person who does my alterations can transform anything from a chiffon gown to a tweed suit and, when I was last there, he was converting a pair of snakeskin trousers into a skirt. Complete size reductions and enhancements are his speciality and he can work on most fabrics, including leather, suede and sheepskin. Find out who's the best in your town by asking the top designer shops who they use for their customer alterations.

Part Four
Attitude

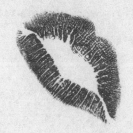

The question everyone always wants to know about girls in glamorous careers is do they use their sexuality to get to the top? Well I don't know about Hollywood, but I can categorically say that in modelling the 'casting couch' does not exist as a stepping stone from model to supermodel.

Every supermodel I spoke to said that flaunting her sexuality – off the catwalk and away from the camera – was unnecessary and unhealthy because it attracted the wrong energy back. The truth is that these girls don't need to 'put out' because they have other qualities that take them right to the top.

The girls who become superstars aren't always the most beautiful – but they are the girls who've found a good level of confidence and self-esteem, who can take reproof and also accept valid criticism when necessary. They are also the most determined, disciplined and resilient. Getting to the top takes drive. Staying there is the true test of a girl's character.

17
How to make it to the top

A top model will be highly paid and have a glamorous lifestyle, but careers are often short-lived and pressures on the individual are staggeringly high. Remember that becoming a model means becoming a commodity. Performing to the expectations of those employing you and satisfying the demands of a fickle public (who iconise and demonise at whim) requires a personality with a unique temperament and good coping mechanisms.

It also involves an ability to make your own luck. Tests show that when confronted with pressures and problems, people fall into two groups, 'internalists' and 'externalists'. The former group are optimists, extroverts and risk takers who analyse, act and learn from life's difficulties. They believe there is a connection between them and what happens to them and they make their own luck by taking more chances and meeting people who might help them make their dreams come true.

But 'externalists' believe that they have no control over their fate and just let life wash over them, seeing themselves as unlucky and convinced from an early age they will fail. Their passivity seals their fate.

Research recently showed us that children who appeared smiling in school photos were much happier three decades later than unsmiling children, proving the propensity to happiness and an optimistic nature starts young and endures a lifetime.

You **can** make your own good luck with the right outlook and your personality **will** influence how you are treated by fate.

Determination
....

Jerry Hall is a fine example of a positive attitude overcoming childhood adversity. Her father was a brutal man who terrorised Jerry, her mother and four sisters. The last to leave home, thinking her father might kill her if she stayed, Jerry began modelling at 14, and at 15 went to Paris to try to find work and get as far away from her violent, alcoholic father as possible.

'I never thought I was pretty, but I thought I had the right bone structure to make a model. I read every book, memorised every modelling pose and decided modelling was less about being good-looking and more to do with knowing how you would look through the lens, being able to

catch the right light and having total control over every muscle in your face. All of which I taught myself to do.'   *Jerry Hall*

Working long hours, often non-stop till the early morning, when she first arrived in Paris, she willed herself to be successful, because she says she never wanted to be forced to go back home. She's now been a high-earning supermodel for 30 years.

Discipline

'Success for me as a model was down to discipline. The reason I was doing all right was because I got stuck in, and when I had to be in New York I was. There were lots of girls who were going to do very well, but they refused to go to New York because of their dog, or their boyfriend, or whatever.' *Camilla Rutherford*

A unique thing happened in the eighties when the top girls started to become more famous than the products and designers they promoted. Cindy Crawford, Linda Evangelista, Helena Christensen, Elle Macpherson, Claudia Schiffer, Christy Turlington, Naomi Campbell and then Kate Moss were the first models to become multi-national enterprises. This also made them as famous and iconised as most of Hollywood's leading female stars.

Cindy Crawford was the Revlon girl for 11 years and the

first model to make fitness videos, as well as appearing on over 500 magazine covers. Cindy's facial mole (airbrushed out of her first cover of *British Vogue*) and curvaceous figure could have scored against her but simply made her more determined.

> *'I think the public could relate to my mole and my female shape. But I was also successful because I was professional. If it was between me and another girl who might not show up, because she had 'food poisoning' — well they'd give it to me.'* **Cindy Crawford**

Cindy's humble background – her father was an electrician – gave her the drive to succeed financially, and made her more interested in money than in partying. 'I was very conservative with money. Every year I would say to my accountant, "This is probably my best year, so don't let me spend too much"'. Cindy is now worth over $60 million.

Unlike the sporting world, models are not protected by a string of advisers. Apart from Twiggy, models have never had personal managers, making do with an agent they share with many other models. There is no contract between agent and model, which often leaves the girls to make important career decisions for themselves.

> *'Even in my day, the girls who got to the top were smart, as well as understanding how to project themselves in front of the camera. My agency took the credit for my success, but actually I*

was the one who refused to do terrible jobs for bathroom fittings and so on, because I knew they wouldn't enhance my career.'

Fiona Campbell-Walter

Resilience

Supermodels are known for their professionalism in a tough world. New York photographer, John Fisher puts it this way, 'They live the life. Models don't "try" fashion – fashion tries them. It's hard, and it's supposed to be hard. That's what makes it great.'

'The paradox', he says 'is that the great models make it look easy. Their skill is that they make incredible levels of beauty seem attainable to every woman with a credit card.' The truth is, of course, a little different.

Modelling isn't brain surgery but it is a damn sight harder than it looks. Making commercials is particularly tricky because there's more financial risk. Instead of delivering one perfect frame from a thousand shots (as in stills photography) a model has to deliver 25 perfect frames for every second of film.

A great model knows nearly as much about the camera as the photographer, certainly where her most flattering angles are and where the lens is looking. Her timing and movements have to be perfect and she must look as though it's all done without a second thought. Every re-take costs serious money, so a model with an overall understanding of how to deliver the goods is always in demand.

Flexibility

• •

Some days you're the butterfly, some days you're the windscreen ...

Kate Moss has a reputation for always giving her best and turning in a master performance even from a difficult brief. She's known to be courteous, persistent and flexible.

Flexibility is crucial for most jobs as it allows you to tolerate a fair amount of ups and downs and to constructively and easily adapt to change. In fact, flexibility can turn challenging situations into amazing opportunities.

TIP If you hit a tricky situation, imagine yourself on an unsinkable raft. No matter how rough the sea, the raft will always float. You can feel safe and secure because you're unsinkable.

Kate is also hugely popular with photographers because she's fun to work with and totally unaffected. Provided she's got what she needs to do her job, she treats those around her as equals and always makes the time to say goodbye to everyone personally, even after a late exhausting shoot.

Solid self-esteem

• •

Linda Evangelista is popular with photographers for different reasons. She has a reputation as a perfectionist and has been known to make normally fearless film crews quake in her presence. She simply wants to do her best and always delivers her side of the bargain – polished, product-selling perfection. A true professional.

Linda lets it be known that she values herself and when you value yourself you treat your own needs as important. If something's wrong, you sort it out because you know you're worth it. Healthy self-esteem makes you feel happy and proud of your achievements whilst you continue to work on those areas of your personality that need improving.

How to look assertive even if you don't feel it

- Keep your head straight – tilting it makes you appear vulnerable.

- Take a deep breath before speaking. It gives you time to think, relaxes you and lowers your voice a tone, making you sound more authoritative.

- Look people in the eye.

- Give yourself an assertive expression by freezing your face as you breathe in.

- Stand up straight, pull in your stomach, tuck your buttocks in, lift your chest and keep your shoulders back and down.

- Research tells us only 7% of meaning is carried in the words you choose, 55% is carried in your body language and the rest in the tone of your voice

> **TIP** It takes 21 days to establish a habit. If you keep up your assertive behaviour for three weeks without slipping, you'll have cracked it

Supermodel motivation

Jerry Hall has always taken responsibility for her life and constantly finds new ways to motivate herself by setting goals she wants and needs to achieve. Whether it's completing an Open University course, writing a first novel, running in a marathon – aiming for and achieving regular targets is important.

'I could lunch with girlfriends, shop and socialise all day but what a complete waste of time...I like to have projects and being creative. As well as acting I'm doing an Open University course in Humanities. Work is important for my self-esteem. It also means I am financially independent and can look after myself.'

Jerry Hall

Twelve ways to get motivated

1. *Set your goal. Make it attainable but challenging and dedicate yourself to reaching it. If you don't have a goal, ask yourself why?*

2. *Be clear about your motivation. Achieving one goal you really want is more satisfying than several you don't feel passionate about.*

3. *Build up your dream. Each week, tell yourself you're a little closer to the target.*

4. *Never settle for second place. You want to be the best.*

5. *Take a day off if you get over-tired. Pushing it is counter-productive.*

6. *Be honest with yourself. If it's not going to plan, ask yourself why. Constructive criticism is vital to progress.*

7. *Learn from your mistakes. Losing can be a useful tool for self-examination.*

8. *Don't expect instant results. Anything worthwhile takes time and effort.*

9. *Be realistic. If you suffer a setback, don't give up. Every failure brings you closer to success.*

10. *Enjoy yourself. If you genuinely love what you're doing, you're almost bound to be good at it.*

11. *Visualise the successful outcome in great detail.*

12. *Judge your performance irrespective of results. Even if you're highly successful, ask yourself if you did your best. Could you have improved any areas?*

Have a clear focus about your goals but never be TOO pleased with yourself when you achieve them. Fate has a peculiar way of bringing you down to earth when you don't do it yourself.

18

Understanding stress levels to help you cope better

The girls who stay at the top have good strategies for handling stress. This is because they recognise that life isn't about the events thrown at them, but how they handle those experiences that counts. They know it's the meaning they give to events that causes stress, not the events themselves.

Approaching each day with a positive attitude and seeking out pleasant situations, rather than crisis or conflict, is essential for a model's well being. She knows she looks a thousand times better when her face is not pinched, worried, pale and intense, and she knows she's less likely to smoke, drink, over/under eat, and more likely to have a happy relationship when she uses sensible mechanisms for coping with pressure.

Stress is an emotive and misunderstood subject. It's

important to understand that you can be healthy and happy and still suffer from the stresses of everyday living. We can't make life run smoothly all the time, so sometimes all we can do is damage limitation. Remember that having a lot to do is not the same as being stressed.

TIP A few drops of Bach Rescue Remedy or Star of Bethlehem tincture infused in a glass of water and sipped slowly, really does help keep anxiety at bay.

Everyone suffers from stress in varying degrees, but it doesn't have to be negative. Pressure can be a powerful, stimulating motivator, urging us to achieve certain goals in our lives. But when pressure exceeds our ability to cope, then it becomes stress.

The important thing is to recognise the different types of stress and to identify negative stress before it becomes harmful.

Stress used to be the word we used in conjunction with major situations – bereavement, serious illness, divorce, job loss. These days we classify all irritating situations as stressful – waiting at airports; not having the right outfit; queuing at the supermarket. We tend to exaggerate 'awful' things in our lives. It's easy to say that motorways make us panic or computers make us nervous, but it's not the computer that's making us nervous, it's how we react to it.

> ⭐ **TIP** Drinking alcohol on an empty stomach can exaggerate feelings of stress, partly because it gives a feeling of losing control, and when you're already struggling to keep things together, it simply makes things worse. So if you fancy a tipple, wait until you've eaten.

It helps to understand that there are three different categories for stress:

1. Pressure, which is usually a positive stress because it's motivating – like finishing a report on time.

2. Stress from daily annoyances – delayed flights and computer crashes. It's frustrating but soon forgotten. Everyday stresses like these can often be overcome by planning. Simple remedies like choosing tomorrow's outfit the night before rather than when eating breakfast, or charging your mobile phone regularly so you don't become incommunicado if you're running late.

3. More serious situations like losing someone or something close to you, severe illness or financial ruin.

Stress-busting superfoods

- *Wholemeal bread, cereals, pasta. Rich in vitamin B to help the nervous system.*
- *Brightly coloured fruit & vegetables. Helps boost the immune system because they are packed with disease-fighting phyto-nutrients.*

- *Herbal teas (Camomile, Lemon Balm). Relaxing and soothing before bed.*
- *Other stress-busting foods include: Artichoke, Beans, Borage, Broccoli, Cabbage, Carrots, Grapefruit, Lavender, Lemon Balm, Lentils, Mango, Muesli, Nuts, Oats, Oranges, Papaya, Rice, Strawberries.*

The five-part stress buster

1. Assess It. Rate the amount of stress you're feeling on a scale of one to ten. Then rate the importance of that situation on a scale of one to ten, where ten is serious injury or worse. When you've missed a bus, your stress might be seven when the importance of the situation is really only a two, so you're creating your own unnecessary stress.

2. See The Big Picture. When you're stressed, picture yourself in three months time. Will the problem be as stressful as it is now or will you almost be laughing at it? Normally it will be forgotten in a few weeks, or even days.

3. Get A Handle On It. If you think you've had a disastrous day, take time to watch the news and discover what real tragedy is.

4. Solve It. Don't waste time on the problem – spend time finding the solution. Think expansively rather than narrowly. There are more options than you think.

5. Don't Worry. It won't make it better or worse. Worrying is
    a habit from childhood and is simply superstitious thinking
    most of the time.

How to calm down

Learning how to seriously relax is the way to true beauty.
We live in exciting times where a challenging and hectic
lifestyle is seen as a reflection of professional and social
status. We work hard and our spare time is used for exercise
or domestic duties. We barely stop for breath and at times
it's easy to forget there is life outside work – it seems to run
our lives rather than the other way round.

TIP Shaking your hands vigorously from the wrists has
an instant calming effect

Even if your head believes you can thrive on continuous
stress, your body will eventually tell you otherwise. The
body needs to experience pleasure and satisfaction to stay
healthy and happy. Holidays and weekends off are not a
luxury; they're an investment in your health for life.

It's vital to incorporate play into your life – enjoying a
relaxed non-pressure activity that allows you to be creative
and have fun. Vigorous exercise at the gym is good for
letting off steam, but it's not playing. Watching a film,

reading a book (not about work) romping with children and pets, and visiting an art gallery is playing.

Then there's totally relaxing, where you try to make at least 20 minutes a day completely yours. Take a long relaxing bath or simply sit in silence and enjoy the moment – but you must do it alone.

Chilling

You can **meditate** simply by focusing your breathing. Your brain will absorb the rhythm and quieten down. Feel the air as it enters your nostrils and moves down to fill your lungs completely.

If you're finding it very hard to unwind try **visualisation**. This is so easy – footballers do it before a match. Imagine you're in the perfect holiday location – a beach, in the mountains, by the sea, in a meadow of flowers. Include all your senses in your holiday image – sight, sound, touch, taste and smell.

If you're imagining yourself on a beach, really smell the salty water as it laps the shore, feel the warmth of the sun on your skin, hear the lapping of the waves and watch the fronds of palm trees waving above you. You will feel calmer in minutes. Stay in this frame of mind for as long as it feels good.

Regular **massages** are a great way to relax, especially massages using calming aromatherapy oils such as lavender. A good massage makes you feel indulged and pampered, improves your circulation, relieves knotted muscles and balances your mind.

Book one now instead of having a manicure or drink with the girls – or better still book a masseur to come to your home. It may appear to be the ultimate luxury, but massage is extremely beneficial and money very well spent.

Prepare yourself for any event mentally and physically with an **aromatherapy bath**. Simply dip the lights, put on soft music, light a candle and add three to five drops of essential oil to a warm bath.

- For an exhausted brain – patchouli, basil or peppermint

- For terrible nerves – lavender, sage, basil, jasmine

- For resentment – rose oil

- For low confidence – camomile or jasmine

- For grumpiness – lavender, camomile, marjoram

> 'A hot bath makes me feel good, especially with a new discovery of mine — amazing oils by the Oils of Roseberry Company which are hand-blended in Thailand.'　　　**Liberty Ross**

Sleep

If you're over-excited or know you're not going to be able to sleep, put a few drops of lavender oil on a tissue near your pillow, drink some camomile tea and do some yoga breathing:

- Lie on the floor with your legs stretched out and your arms at your side with the palms facing up.

- Draw breath in through your nose, down your throat and out again. As you inhale, your stomach should swell and deflate as you exhale.

- Repeat several times.

The eight steps to good sleep

1. Realise that sleep is the best natural form of stress relief.

2. Make sure your bedroom is relaxing – designed solely for the purpose of sleep – no television or computer.

3. Darkness is crucial as strong light interferes with the body's production of the hormone melatonin, which is essential for sleep. Invest in black-out curtains or a sleep-mask.

4. Never over-heat the bedroom – it causes restlessness.

5. Avoid caffeine after 4 pm.

6. Never exercise in the evening – it pumps the body full of adrenaline, which will keep you awake.

7. Avoid rich foods at night – your body will be digesting not resting.

8. If you can't sleep after 30 minutes get up and do something. Otherwise bed becomes a reminder of sleeplessness.

'Getting the right amount of sleep every night would have to be my best beauty secret. I look better, feel better and seem to radiate more happiness when I've had lots of sleep.'

Catherine Hurley

19

Knowing the difference between disease and dis-ease

We all recognise the infuriating work colleague who never seems to be around to help take the load when work is at its most pressurised – she's caught a cold again and thinks it's 'best not to pass on the germs'.

Somehow she makes a miraculous recovery by the weekend and can't wait to tell you all about her Saturday night antics on Monday morning. Well, the modelling world is no different.

When a model looks as though she has the potential to make it to the top, her agency will assess her 'staying power'. Not in terms of commercial popularity, but in her ability to be totally reliable – to stay the course.

'There is no set formula for success as a model, but certain character traits, like laziness, are best avoided. Also, you spend so much time travelling as a model it's important to be happy in your own company.

'There is no pressure if you plan your schedules well and think ahead. I give myself enough time and space to plan my life at a pace that makes me happy and feels comfortable, and I make sure I keep my weekends free.'

Catherine Hurley

Every model agency in the world has had a girl on their books who appears to get 'sick' more often than normal and usually before an important job. Her headaches, tummy upsets and colds are regular occurrences; her bathroom cupboards overflow with potions and pills and she's always the one with food intolerances ('I can't touch wheat and dairy') but she thinks nothing of getting totally wrecked at a bar.

Getting real

The truth is she uses her body's 'ailments' to disguise her mental fear of failure. Blaming her body for letting her down allows her to offset and deny the reality of her predicament, which is her lack of self-esteem and her fear of not living up to expectations.

Quite often this type of girl is also a bad timekeeper, but it is never her fault, e.g. 'I can't help it if the taxi was slow'.

And she will always rationalise her unreliability, e.g. 'I didn't really want the job anyway', or 'I'll show them' in a bizarre embodiment of self-deluding arrogance.

Tackling the problem of feeling unworthy can simply be a question of becoming less self-obsessed and taking more responsibility for her life, or she may need professional help in dealing with her issues.

She's the girl a photographic team don't need on a complicated location shoot. They want 'one of the boys' who can lug a suitcase into the jungle, change behind a bush, knock up a sandwich, make the photographer laugh, the client swoon, suggest the answer to a lighting problem and photograph like an angel. She may have a headache, she might even have a slight cold, but guess what – no-one will ever know.

Spend time with supportive people

When I was at the height of my modelling career, I went to a dinner party given by a married couple who knew my, then, boyfriend. The hostess introduced me to the other guests by saying, 'This is Vikki, everybody. She's a muddle – ooh sorry I mean a model, ha, ha'. After she'd referred to me in this way four or five times during the evening, my boyfriend whispered, 'Don't worry, she's cross because you earn ten times more than her husband and you're half his age'.

The hostess hadn't given me a chance; she had a preconceived impression of me based on her resentment. Of course, I didn't realise it then and kept wondering how I'd upset her and thinking it must be all my fault.

It's inevitable that many women, especially financially independent, successful women will run into envy and scorn some time during their lives. The trick is to actively avoid negative influences and spend as much time as possible with supportive people who make you feel good and as little time as possible with those who make you feel uncomfortable or 'wrong'.

Sift through your family and friends and assess honestly who is good for you and who isn't. If you must spend time with someone who drains or upsets you, reduce the amount of time you are ever together.

TIP Realise that people who are genuinely happy don't need to constantly put down, ridicule or criticise others.

On a more serious level, if you feel another person has severely damaged you psychologically (there is a particularly fine-tuned form of intimate, persistent and highly articulate mental cruelty that can go almost unnoticed in relationships) then it's not a bad idea to visit a recommended therapist and sort out your feelings on the matter. And then you can move on.

If you've been damaged financially or physically and you feel it appropriate and important, call the person who damaged you into account through the legal system. After that you must move on otherwise you are inflicting damage upon yourself.

You won't ever regret severing these negative ties and you'll allow much more room in your life for happiness.

Gratitude

Time rushes by so quickly that we tend to ignore or take for granted the good things in our lives and focus on the parts that slow us down like relationship hiccups or work pressures. We don't stop to think how lucky we are to be healthy and to have such freedom of choice in all areas of our lives.

It was only when I looked back on my modelling career, for the purpose of this book, that I realised how lucky I was to be given the opportunity to change and develop so many aspects of my life through modelling.

At school I grew up with the miserable nicknames of 'hat-stand' and 'lamp-post' and detested my gangly body more than anything on earth. I longed to be like my petite, voluptuous best friend and used to pray that I would shrink in my sleep. That I went on to make a substantial living for ten years from the very thing I hated most is a strange irony not lost on me now.

Regularly traversing the world alone as a model before I was barely out of my teens (was I really that intrepid?) is something I took entirely for granted, together with the weird and wonderful people I met along the way.

The sheer pleasure of knowing two of the most legendary fashion editors of all time, *American Vogue's* Diana Vreeland ('Never wear hats, my dear, they don't suit your head') and *Italian Vogue's* Anna Piaggi ('Always wear hats, sweetie, they balance your big chin') and of discovering the different cultures and similar kindness of the people whose countries I worked in, now makes me feel privileged and ever grateful.

20

The key to happiness

The greatest beautifiers in the world are happiness and good health. A wonderful smile and boundless energy are far more attractive – whatever the owner's physique – than a miserable, pinched face above a tense body. There are many areas we can't change about our lives, but there are things we can do to be happier right now.

Give out

Care about other people. It's an important part of happiness to give something back to the community if the system's been good to you. Supermodel Christy Turlington has always tried to look beyond the 'micro' of her admittedly privileged life by doing community service and volunteer work. She strongly believes that helping other people heals her and finds it 'life enhancing'.

She finds her charity work so rewarding that she recently set up a Manhattan office in which she can hatch ideas for future projects. She has also formed The Christy Turlington Foundation, an organisation for a myriad of good works, ranging from an anti-smoking campaign to working on behalf of UNICEF in Afghanistan.

Opening up your horizons allows you to be aware of those less fortunate than yourself and gives you the simple, pure pleasure of helping to re-balance the odds in life.

Get closer to the people you love

Being loved and knowing how to love back are the fundamental basics of true happiness. Talk about your feelings with the ones you love. Good communication skills are vital if we want to keep our relationships happy and stress-free. The best partnerships don't have huge conflicts because both parties have learned it's essential to communicate openly and in an appropriate way – not only in a crisis but also in everyday life.

> *I'm very lucky in that I come from a very close family and my background gave me the ability to enjoy and understand those close to me. I can separate those who want something from me from those who genuinely care for me. My joy in life is my son — I want him to grow up with the love and support I had from my own parents.'*
> *Helena Christensen*

You'll also be happier if you don't expect your partner or future partner to be the answer to all your problems.

Another person, however wonderful, can't make you happy. A good partnership is about companionship and trust, not unrealistically high expectations that few people could ever live up to.

Keep smiling

Make yourself laugh even if you don't feel like it. Laughter triggers the release of feel-good hormones from your brain, which improve your mood, boosts your immune system, helps you relax and reduces pain.

Much of our happiness depends on how we relate to ourselves – how much we're in tune with our needs and how skilfully we utilise our inner resources to keep ourselves positive and optimistic.

You'll know you're on the right track when you naturally laugh and smile often and when little things make you happy. It's worth remembering that the more fun you have in life, the more fun you are to be with.

Be assertive

Don't be afraid to ask for what you want and saying 'no' when you don't want.

Many of us find it extremely hard to say 'no' directly to requests, but it is essential for your happiness and well-being to allow people to know your boundaries.

This is all about valuing yourself and treating your own

needs as important. You are telling people that your time and place in this world is as justified as theirs. Practise saying 'no' in front of the mirror – it gets easier!

> '*Modelling has taught me to stand up for myself. I've become much more assertive when choosing my modelling jobs. I've learned to say "no" with grace, in a way that doesn't upset people, which I wasn't very good at before.*'
>
> Catherine Hurley

Set attainable goals

Make a list of goals you need to achieve, and give yourself a realistic timescale for making them happen. You can achieve what you want as long as you go about it in the right way.

Begin with your goal in mind and picture the scene of your success. Write down a definite plan of what you want and refer to it regularly to check your progress and what you still need to do to succeed.

> '*It's important for me to have professional goals in my life, as well as having a happy home life. My photography is important to me and I'm putting together an exhibition of my work, which includes recent fashion photography for "Vogue" and "Dazed and Confused".*'
>
> Helena Christensen

Be prepared to overcome inevitable obstacles, by reassuring yourself that you will conquer any problem and triumph. Don't be nervous when you approach your goal. Get to know the unique satisfaction of pushing your own boundaries, and discover what makes you tick when you're really challenged. If you suffer a setback, realise that every failure brings you closer to success and learn from the experience.

Face problems

Always look for constructive solutions. Never live in the problem itself. This calls for positive living through positive thinking and the realisation that worry doesn't change a thing. As long as you keep looking for positive solutions, keep an open mind about the way the solutions present themselves and don't give up, you'll find a way through.

Make clear plans for resolving your problems and have the confidence to implement the necessary changes needed for more peace of mind – and to allow other people to be as they want to be. You cannot control their actions or thoughts.

Remember you cannot make life run smoothly all the time. Sometimes you have to accept that things are out of your control, accept this calmly, then you've done your best. As William James said, 'The art of being wise is the art of knowing what to overlook'.

Practise moderation

Do a bit of everything that agrees with you. **Never become obsessive about diet, exercise or beauty regimes.** Your outlook should be self-maintenance rather than self-obsession. If you spend a fortune pampering yourself, it will all be wasted if you feel worthless inside. External luxuriating does not heal internal problems or loneliness.

Aim to feel rich emotionally by being more in touch with your feelings. Grow to like yourself a lot more and you'll find you'll relate to others in a better way.

Relax

Rest is essential for happy, healthy living. Try to have a regime for 20 minutes at the end of every day to help you unwind – a set yoga routine, reading the evening newspaper, a bath. Realise that this time to yourself is as important as the other areas of your busy life.

Test your serenity rating at the end of the day by seeing if you can sit still without doing anything – simply feeling calm and content – for five minutes. If not, take yourself off for a massage, have an aromatherapy bath, go for a gentle walk or make yourself a cup of herbal tea and read a relaxing book.

Get close to nature

It's the most effective blues-beater there is. Watching animals and birds, appreciating beautiful scenery and clean air and the sun has the same anti-depressant quality as medication. It helps us to get a sense of harmony and balance back into our lives.

Tuning into nature is as important as tuning into our own feelings and our physical needs because it opens our eyes to a level beyond the physical, mental and emotional levels of existence. It helps us to go that one step further and explore the spiritual side of our natures.

Explore the spiritual

Finding a set of values and a sense of life that has meaning and direction will make you happier. You can be spiritual without having any religion. The spiritual side of life is an appreciation of the process of life itself that leads us beyond the purely personal. All you need to access your spiritual side is openness and a sense of curiosity.

Spirituality is very real and in many ways quite ordinary. If you've ever, for example, felt blissfully happy for a moment in time without any obvious reason, had your breath taken away by a spectacular view, marvelled at the close-up intricacy of a plant or flower, felt a special atmosphere in a particular place, then you have experienced the extra-sensory – a very marked inner feeling that cannot be attributed to any of our 'normal' senses.

'If there is one thing I learned from my life as a model it is that beauty is never skin deep and a

girl must develop other areas in order to be an interesting human being.'

Fiona Campbell-Walter

Spiritual experiences touch the very centre of our being – the human soul. To be happy we need to be regularly in touch with our soul, as it helps support and nurture all other aspects of our life.

Connecting with our soul helps to complete the four parts that make up the self – the physical, mental, emotional and spiritual – which work harmoniously together for us to experience complete and total inner happiness.

'My philosophy for a happy life is to feel content inside. Always have new interests in life and don't get too wrapped up in yourself. After all, to be an interesting person you have to be an interested person. A good sense of humour is very, very important and not to be too hard on yourself. The most important thing to realise is that beauty is meaningless if it's self-serving. True beauty really does come from inside.'

Helena Christensen

From the skin to the soul

Be sure to nurture your health and happiness, try things you've never tried before, never stop believing in your dreams – and make sure you die young as late as possible.

I hope the contents of this book have guided and helped you in all the areas that make up the beautiful **you**. All the supermodels who have generously contributed to this book, believe them to be the true beauty secrets of life, as do I.

> *'There's only one universe that you can be certain of improving, and that's your own self.'*
> *Aldous Huxley*

Resources

Fashion websites

The most wonderful life-saving, comprehensive fashion website ever invented, which brings you last season's discounted clothes from every top designer in the world, is
http://www.yoox.com

Get a feel for what's hot and what's not by checking out the best reference websites. Fashion shows are shown as they happen on:
http://www.style.com
http://www.vogue.com
http://www.fashion.net
with backstage shots of models getting ready and every single outfit from the show on the cat-walk, enabling you to plan next season's wardrobe well in advance.

Want the buzz of buying from the hottest boutiques in the world without having to leave home? Go straight to

http://www.net-a-porter.com where stylist and boutique owner Natalie Massenet chooses her favourite seasonal collection pieces from leading designers. Each item is clearly displayed, and, alarmingly for the weak-willed, the site offers sameday messenger service to customers in London and your goodies arrive in a super-chic black gift box.

UK Favourites

Facialists
Jo Malone
Tel: +44 (0)20 7491 9104

Crystal Clear Oxygen Facial
Tel: +44 (0)870 593 493

Teeth whitening
The Britesmile System
Tel: +44 (0)800 0768 769

Trichologist
Philip Kingsley
54 Green Street
London W1K 6RU
Tel: +44 (0)20 7629 4004

Hair Salon
Real
8 Cale Street
London SW3 3QU
Tel: +44 (0)20 7589 0877
Website: http://www.realhair.co.uk

Perfumeries
L'Artisan Parfumeur
17 Cale Street
London SW3
Tel: +44 (0)20 7352 4196

Les Senteurs
227 Ebury Street
London SW1
Tel: +44 (0)20 7730 2322

Cosmetic surgery adviser
Wendy Lewis
Tel: +44 (0)20 7828 8244
Website: http://www.wlbeauty.com

Skin-brush
Revital
Website: http://www.revital.com

Alterations genius
Tosca Tassoun at First Tailoring
85 Lower Sloane Street
London SW1
Tel: +44 (0)20 7730 1400

Australian Favourites

....

Spa
Spa Chakra
The Finger Wharf
Wooloomooloo
Sydney
Tel: +61 (0)2 9368 0888

Hair Salons
Joh Bailey
Shop 30
Chifley Plaza
Sydney
Tel: +61 (0)2 223 7673

Adroit
241 Bridge Road
Richmond
Melbourne 3122
Tel: +61 (0)3 428 1706

Teeth Whitening
The Laserbrite System
Dr Mark Casiglia
59 Burns Bay Road
Lane Cove
Sydney 2006
Tel: +61 (0)2 9427 1623

Alterations

Your Expert Service
Little Collins Street
Melbourne
Tel: +61 (0)3 3221 5994

Hang Out
Leichhardt
Sydney
Tel: +61 (0)2 9572 6477

Designer Shoe Repairs

Rekaris
Lonsdale Street
Melbourne
Tel: +61 (0)3 9669 4669

Subiaco Shoe Maker
Perth
Tel: +61 (0)8 9381 2749

Chifley Shoe Worx
Sydney
Tel: +61 (0)2 9223 9670

Cosmetic surgery advice

The Cosmetic Surgery Clinic
Sydney
Website: http://www.cosmeticsurgeryoz.com

New Zealand Favourites

Fashion
FashioNZ
Website: http://www.fashionz.co.nz/designer_clothes.htm

Hair Salon
Ginger Megs
7 Albans Street
Merivale
Christchurch
Tel: +64 (3) 355 9276

Cosmetics/Perfumes
Smith and Caughey's
Queen Street
Auckland
Tel: +64 (9) 377 4770

Cosmetic surgery advice
The New Zealand Foundation for Cosmetic Plastic
Surgery
P.O.Box 47 682
Ponsonby
Website: http://nzcosmeticsurgery.org.nz

South African Favourites

Hair Salons
Carlton Hair International
Shop 5, The Place
Cavendish Square
Claremont
Cape Town
Tel: +27 21 61 6877

Burgundy
Shop 105, 1st Level
Sandton Square
Sandton
Johannesberg
Tel: +27 11 884 0192

Massage
The Chelsea Health and Beauty Clinic
17 Wolfe Street
Wynberg
Cape Town
Tel: +27 21 797 6754

Elaine Brennan
6 North Park Centre
3rd Avenue
Parktown North
Johannesburg
Tel: +27 11 788 5213

Index